TOUGH DECISIONS
IN CARE OF
ELDERLY **LOVED** ONES

Dignity | Safety | Quality Of Life

A Guide For Caregivers

Mahesh Moolani, MD

Copyright © 2020
Mahesh Moolani, MD
Tough Decisions
In Care of Elderly Loved Ones
Dignity | Safety | Quality Of Life
A Guide For Caregivers

www.elderlylovedones.com

All rights reserved.

No part of this publication may be reproduced, distributed, or transmitted in any form or by any means, including photocopying, recording, or other electronic or mechanical methods, without the prior written permission of the publisher, except in the case of brief quotations embodied in critical reviews and certain other non-commercial uses permitted by copyright law.

Mahesh Moolani, MD

Printed in the United States of America
First Printing 2020
First Edition 2020
ISBN: 978-1-7344077-1-6

10 9 8 7 6 5 4 3 2 1

Cover design by Premium Digital Marketing
Graphics by Premium Digital Marketing

Disclaimer:

Please note that all the patient stories described are loosely based on real life encounters. Whilst the issues are and some conversations are taken from real encounters, I have endeavored to anonymize any identifiable information.

Although the author has made every effort to ensure that the information in this book was correct at press time, the author does not assume and hereby disclaim any liability to any party for any loss, damage, or disruption caused by errors or omissions, whether such errors or omissions result from negligence, accident, or any other cause. The author has used multiple sources as references, which are listed at the end of the book. These information from these sources will not be clearly tied to the end of book references.

This book is not intended as a substitute for the medical advice of your own health care advisor. The reader should regularly consult a doctor in matters relating to his/her health and particularly with respect to any symptoms that may require diagnosis or medical attention.

Dedicated to my paternal grandmother Godhawari and in memory of my maternal grandmother Bhomi.

Special thanks to:

My parents Hotchand and Pushpa,

wife Urmila,

siblings Ishwari, Kailash, and Javanty and their spouses Ramesh, Janta and Prem, respectively,

and sons Harsh and Satya, who all inspire me to do what I love.

Acknowledgment

I am thankful to the following people who helped me edit the book.

Thomas Lovett
Tim Thompson
Vera Hanson
Carroll Laswell
Kathy Lewis
Mukesh Desai
Harsh Moolani
and
Kirsten Rees

Table of Contents

Introduction 1
Empathy and Patience 5
Living Will or Advance Directives or Advance Care Planning 9
Home Health Services and Non-Medical Home Help 13
Personal Care Homes 19
Skilled Nursing Facilities - Specialized Medical Services 23
Palliative Care: A Specialized Medical Approach 27
Hospice: Caring For the Terminally Ill 31
Part I: Mental conditions of the elderly loved ones 37
    Depression 39
    Anxiety 47
    Dementia 55
Part II: Health of the elderly loved ones 67
    Heart Disease 69
    Lung Conditions 73
    Cancer 79
    Neurological Disorders 83
Part III: Physical condition of the elderly loved ones 89
    Physical Condition and Daily Living 91
    Medications 113
Part IV: Overall financial and social conditions of the caregivers 123
    Factors Caretakers Must Consider About Themselves 125
    What to Look For 135
Further Reading: 137
Connect with MD Mahesh Moolani: 138
References 139

Introduction

What are the tough decisions for elderly loved ones

There are many decisions to be made with and on the behalf of our loved ones as they age. It can be an emotional time and often these decisions need to be made based on what is best for them, rather than what we want to do for practical or financial reasons.

Often these decisions are made under the most difficult of circumstances and through necessity rather than choice. This book will cover many of the situations and decisions we may need to consider and provides answers in a clear and simple way with empathy and understanding.

In 1960, the World Bank calculated that the average American could expect to live just under seventy years. That life expectancy has slowly grown since then; the average life expectancy in the US is upwards of seventy-eight years old. While families have been able to celebrate and enjoy time with loved ones longer, this expansion of life expectancy can take a toll as well. As our loved ones live longer, disease has increased opportunity to create challenges in their lives.

Older adults may find themselves struggling to accomplish tasks which were easy five years, one year, or maybe even six months ago. Many elderly people want to maintain their independence even though they no longer can drive, cook, mow the lawn or even go to the bathroom alone. Even those who are wheelchair-bound still may seek some measure of independence. But advance planning and good communication can help prepare families for difficult transitions.

Common difficult situations families with elderly loved ones face include:

1. Telling a loved one they should no longer drive
2. Medical treatment in the face of a poor prognosis
3. Placement in an assisted living, personal care, or skilled nursing facility
4. Discontinuing certain medications, which the family thinks are necessary
5. Removal of guns from a home (where relevant)
6. Advance care planning, including decisions about which, if any, life-sustaining efforts should be made
7. Seeking palliative or hospice care
8. Financial planning

These decisions are extremely difficult and can polarize families. Many, if not all of them, are inevitable as we age. Thinking about these issues in advance, hearing their wishes, discussing with friends and family can ease their burden and ensure they receive the level of care desired.

This book is divided into four categories:

1. Mental condition of the elderly patient
2. Health of the elderly patient
3. Physical condition of the elderly patient
4. Overall financial and social conditions of the caregivers

Given the intricacies of caring for the elderly, these issues cannot be addressed individually; a more holistic approach is needed. We cannot try to help an elderly relative with a physical issue without taking their mental health and the impact on caregivers into account.

As we discuss decision-making and elder care, there are three criteria we need to keep in mind:

1. Dignity of the patient
2. Safety of the patient
3. Quality of the patient's life

We will touch on these three criteria numerous times during our discussions, in this book.

Here it must be emphasized that quality of life is not defined by the doctors or other healthcare staff. It has to be defined and determined by the patient and their loved ones.

Empathy and Patience

Empathy

Empathy is more than just loving an elderly loved one. It is more than simply making the decision we may feel is best for our loved one. Empathy is different from sympathy. Empathy means putting ourselves in someone else's shoes and making an informed decision. Empathy is seeing through our loved ones' eyes, hearing through her ears, feeling her emotions and thinking about her thoughts. It requires internalizing her feelings and acting accordingly. It is a crucial component when working with older adults.

As people grow older, they become increasingly vulnerable and their needs increase. This may be for a number of reasons - they don't want to be seen as a burden, feel uncomfortable switching roles having been the caregiver to their children, may be unaware. However, it can be quite difficult for elderly loved ones to show and explain their needs to family and friends. They may try to tackle issues such as financial stress, physical limitations, poor health, or loneliness on their own to avoid "imposing" or "being a burden" to others. This is where empathy comes in. Given that a loved one may be reluctant to ask for help, we must be actively watching and listening for signs of a problem. We must be ready to help, sometimes before help is sought.

In many cases, empathy is the most important thing we can provide. Our loved ones want us to be on their side when they are frail or in distress. They want us to be their strength when they need it most.

This is how we can empathize with elderly loved ones:

- Understand that listening is more important than talking.
- Talk in a soft voice while showing our concern.
- Focus on their feelings and their needs.
- Asking them how they are feeling, if we think anything is wrong.
- Offer to help with the groceries, dishes, laundry or house-cleaning.
- Don't push if an offer of help is refused. Back off, give it a little time and try again with a different approach.

Mary and David, 83 and 85 respectively, have lived in their home alone for last 65 years. They have two children who themselves are in their 60s. Mary recently had a fall, which caused hip fracture. She needed urgent surgery, and after surgery she couldn't walk and needed some rehabilitation at a nursing home. While in a nursing home, she developed pneumonia and became very weak. Despite the best efforts of the rehab team, she didn't recover completely and needed help. David was adamant on taking her home while the nurses, physical therapists, and doctors believed that Mary needed more care than David could have provided. David himself is too old and frail. The son tried to make David understand for few hours but did not have any success. David was furious at his son for being "too bossy and not understanding his feelings". Their daughter, Deborah, sat patiently with them for long hours every day and listened to their concerns. She told them that she "understands their feelings and won't do anything against their wishes". She let them express their frustration and anxiety. Finally, after addressing all the concerns to the best of her ability and according to the wishes of her parents, Deborah convinced them to move to an assisted living facility. Deborah visited the facility with the parents, let them meet the staff, and checked the quality of help the facility provided. She made sure that all their needs would be properly addressed and this is how she was able to convince both her parents.

When we see or sense there is a problem, the first question we need to ask is not "How will I get him or her to accept help?" It should be "How much help do they need?" It's a critical step in the process. If we seek to provide more help than actually needed a loved one may feel we are trying to steal their independence.

Patience

If empathy is seeing through a loved one eyes, patience is accepting what we find when we look. American society is built on speed. We like fast cars, we eat fast food and we rush from meeting to meeting. But as we age, we slow down physically and mental processes may slow as well. This can create tension and stress when, for example, dining with an elderly relative.

If a senior is capable of feeding himself, but does so slowly, allow them to eat slowly rather than offering to feed them. If they can use the bathroom, we don't have to get the toilet paper for them. If they can safely use a walker, allow them to do so, rather than suggest it's time for a wheelchair. If our elderly relative can take care of an issue safely, it's fine to let them do so.

Just be patient.

Showing patience with our loved ones allows them to maintain their dignity. Quality of life and dignity are very important for them and that's why they want to do as many things as they can by themselves. This means that we should not interfere unless their safety is being compromised.

We should only intervene when things become unsafe - when we see that they are having falls, we have to intervene. When dementia, arthritis or other problems impair their ability to drive, we need to intervene. Anything that may threaten their safety should be given the highest priority. But until that point, act with restraint. Remember, even when our loved ones have a threatening disease like dementia, they will still want their independence. We need to let them have their independence for as long as safely possible.

Just be patient and take it easy for the sake of our loved ones and ourselves.

Throughout this book, I will be presenting ideas and tactics to help our loved ones and help us make tough decisions for them while being empathetic and patient.

Every situation is unique; there is no single solution for everyone. So, this book is less about providing solutions than about finding a solution that is best for our situation.

Living Will or Advance Directives or Advance Care Planning

A living will or an advance directive is a document which explains a person's preference of treatment in case of imminent death.

In the simplest sense, these documents help doctor and healthcare providers know what to do if, for example, an elderly loved one's heart stops beating or they stop breathing. Would they want the doctor to do CPR or hook them up to a ventilator to serve as life support? This documentation only becomes valid if and when our elderly loved ones can't communicate their desires and wishes.

Why do it? Why should one make such a document?

Creating a living will allows elderly loved ones to make their own decisions in the most critical stage of their life. By having the power to make the decision beforehand, it will allow them to be in complete control of the way to proceed during tense situations for them and their family.

We have to tell our elderly loves ones "You make this decision, then I will do everything as per your wishes, so I don't have the burden of making that decision'.

When advance care directives are not available, I have seen families fighting while trying to make this decision. Some children want the parent to be resuscitated while others don't, and this causes huge friction among the children at the time when the family should be there to support one another.

When an elderly loved one has made this decision beforehand, this pressure is removed from the family and allows everything to be done according to their preference.

A living will document has three parts:

1. Does one want to have chest compressions and CPR (cardiopulmonary resuscitation) and want to be put on a ventilator (life support machine) if that person can't breathe or if his or her heart stops beating?

    Elderly loved ones can choose to

    a) die naturally or

    b) chose resuscitation

2. In case one can't eat by themselves and can't make their own decisions, do they want to have artificial nourishment and fluids through tube feeding like tube through the nose or mouth or stomach or feeding through their blood vessels?

    Elderly loved ones can choose

    a) tube feeding or

    b) decline tube feeding

3. Do our elderly loved ones want to donate organs?

    They can choose to

    a) donate particular organs or

    b) donate all organs or

    c) decline to donate any organs

Elderly loved ones should fill out this form according to their own personal wishes and after considering their health condition and discussing with their family.

Elderly loved ones will sign and date the form once they have filled out the form in the presence of two witnesses who are over the age of eighteen, OR in the presence of a notary public.

The following people CANNOT be a witness to or serve as a notary public:

- A blood relative
- A person who is going to inherit their property
- An employee of a healthcare facility in which we are a patient (unless the employee serves as a notary public)
- The attending physician
- Any person directly financially responsible for their healthcare.

Some people choose to nominate a "Healthcare surrogate" or "Durable Power of Attorney for Healthcare" or "Healthcare Proxy" who will make their decisions in case of terminal illness or unconsciousness or when they can't communicate.

If our elderly loved one wants to make someone their healthcare surrogate, then they have to make sure that person is at least eighteen years old and that they trust that person to make the correct decision for them. The proxy can't be their doctor unless he is a family member. The elderly loved one does not have to nominate a healthcare surrogate if they don't want to. We don't need a lawyer to make the advanced care directive document. One of the easiest ways to fill out these forms is completing an online form.

Home Health Services and Non-Medical Home Help

Home healthcare is a broad term describing an array of healthcare services provided at a patient's home after an injury or ailment, especially when they are advanced in years. Residential healthcare provides greater convenience at a lesser cost. The best part, however, lies in the efficacy of the services. Home healthcare services are as prompt and helpful as the ones provided at nursing facilities and hospitals. Many insurance companies cover these services.

However, certain aspects of home care, such as anything that is a part of nonmedical care or medication administered at home, are precluded. At times, some of the services are connected to each other.

There are two types of home healthcare

1. Formal Home Healthcare
2. Informal Long-Term Home Care

Formal Home Healthcare

Formal home healthcare is provided by medically trained personnel such as a case management nurse, physical therapist or registered nurse, who performs medical assistance-related tasks for the patient and their family. These tasks are, in most cases, prescribed by physicians and carried out as a part of the patient's therapy. Apart from this, they monitor the health and medication of the patient on a continual basis, making informed and necessary decisions whenever required.

Informal Long-Term Home Healthcare

Informal home healthcare is offered by non-medically skilled senior care helpers, friends and family caregivers acquainted with the basic healthcare needs of the patient. They perform tasks such as watching out for unusual behavior, filling prescriptions and following up on the physician visits. With more people being educated on the perks of informal home healthcare, there has been an increase in people opting for informal long-term home healthcare.

Important Home Care Services include, but are not limited to:

- Physical treatments such as mobility exercises and strengthening;
- Restoration therapy programs that include occupational and physical therapies;
- IV treatments as a part of drug therapies;
- Pain management;
- Keeping track of dietary restrictions and medication dosage;
- Wound care; and
- Occupational therapies for daily activities like bathing and eating.
- Some common benefits of home healthcare services are:
- Provides assistance with physical and occupational therapy for patients during their post-surgery period while staying in their home.
- Schedules visits with skilled nursing experts who provide services and administer therapies within the comfort of the home.
- Provides healthcare with expertise in senior-specific training.
- Brings down the frequency of the patient's visits to the hospital.

- Aids specialized adaptations to the patient's surroundings, thus making it more comfortable, safe and accessible.
- Provides relief to family members from their responsibilities for a while.
- Brings greater affordability compared to the care offered at skilled nursing facilities or a hospital setting.
- Promotes healing, health and overall happiness.
- Takes care of the personal, cultural, financial, medical and emotional requirements of a patient.

Non-Medical In-Home Care

Non-medical caregivers provide assistance to people in need of care through services such as respite care, companionship and personal care. The common duties of these caregivers include:

- Medication reminders
- Dressing and bathing
- Feeding
- Company and errands
- Transportation or walking assistance

Non-medical care can be divided into two main types:

1. Personal Care
2. Companion Care

Nursing assistants who offer personal care are trained to help people with their special and immediate healthcare needs. While most of these providers are certified and state-licensed, the companion caregivers are meant to assist with subtle housekeeping chores, transportation, socialization and meal preparation. They do not have the training required to help with basic care requirements or personal care.

Benefits of Senior Care

Senior care provided in the home varies widely, based on the needs of the patient. In some cases, the need is limited to simple companionship. In others, the client may require personalized home care services and close monitoring. The most common benefits of in-home elderly care are:

- Offers care within the comfort of the patient's home. Most of the elderly loved ones want to stay at home and would love to have help at home. There is no place which is more comforting for them as their own home.
- Promotes healing.
- Allows family and friends flexibility in visiting. There are no regulated "visiting hours."
- Provides an economic alternative compared to care at a nursing facility or hospital. Medicare doesn't allow more than 100 days of skilled care at a nursing home. After that, a patient can must pay the cost, usually more than $200 per day.
- Prevents or postpones a move to a nursing home.
- Reduces chances of re-hospitalization. The home health workers can usually identify the health problems of elderly loved ones earlier and that will help in their care.
- Promotes freedom and independence.
- Special assistance catered to the needs of elderly loved ones.

Disadvantages of Home Healthcare

The biggest disadvantage is that most insurances will not cover 24/7 care and either the caregivers or our loved ones must cover the cost. The care may cost $15-$30 or more per hour. The cost will depend on the level of care being provided and where our loved ones live.

The Primary care doctors can help find the right care for loved ones. They can guide us in the process as well.

Personal Care Homes

Personal Care Homes, or Residential Care Homes, are facilities that offer seniors nursing care and comfort like that of residential homes. The setting of these facilities is small with a homelike appearance. These adult homes come with semi-private and private rooms and are usually run by the actual residents of the property. A personal care home is a smart option when it comes to aiding elderly people in need of daily care but who prefer to share a home with a group of seniors or a family. Mostly licensed, some of these facilities admit and care for seniors with memory impairment or Alzheimer's syndrome.

Services Offered by a Residential Care Home

The exact services offered depend on the residential care that we opt for since it varies with each facility. While some might offer specialized services like field trips and senior aerobics, here are a few amenities offered by most:

- Home cooked meals 1 to 3 times a day, depending on the home;
- Dedicated laundry and housekeeping services;
- Help with activities such as using the restroom, bathing and dressing;
- Social activities and programs; and
- Medical care and management.
- Other services offered:
- Organized outings;
- Shopping trips;

- Transportation facilities to meetings and appointments;
- Movie nights; and
- Company of pets (not common)

A few residential care homes hire personnel meant to care for people with specific needs. For example, a nurse who has been appointed to care for a patient with diabetes will not render generalized services like feeding or bathing them. In some cases, they also aid residents with recommended physical activities and therapies.

Tips to Choose the Right Personal Care Home

Picking the right personal care facility for a loved one is crucial. The internet can help find a facility near us using our area code, region or county. Friends or other family members might offer a recommendation as well. Opting for a licensed home ensures the home undergoes regular inspections and has access to the best service delivery options. Some factors to consider while choosing the right home care facilities are:

<u>Size</u>

A personal care facility may be either small or large. The services offered mostly depend on the lifestyle of the owner and their preferences. Consider whether our loved one prefers larger groups of people or a small-group setting.

<u>Cost</u>

The monthly fees of a personal care facility can range from hundreds to thousands of dollars. While people mostly tend to look for cost-effective options, ensuring that the home has all the required services is also important. Insurance may cover personal care home cost.

Location

Ensure the location is near the residences of family and friends, so they can be convenient in case of emergencies. Proximity to places like churches, libraries and other essential community resources is an added advantage.

Among the steps to take when considering a facility are:

1. Peek into as many rooms as we can.
2. Visit during different hours of the day.
3. Watch how the staff members communicate and interact with the nursing home residents.
4. Ask about the staff qualifications and training.
5. Check out the menu and try a few meals, if possible.
6. Learn about the rules regarding smoking, pets, visitation and other matters.
7. Speak to other residents of the home apart from the administrator and staff.
8. Inquire about additional fees and services offered, if any.

Benefits of a Personal Care Facility

A personal care facility is practically a home away from home for people who feel uncomfortable or do not enjoy staying within a large community. Some common benefits of a personal care facility are:

- A smaller setting allows residents to know each other better.
- Residential care facilities can offer a superior level of personal care.

- Most have staff available round the clock to cater to the needs of residents.
- Tiered levels of care allow seniors to live without personal hassles.

Cost of a Residential Care Facility

The cost of a residential care home is often half that of a nursing home or an assisted living community, although costs may vary with the type and level of care offered. It also depends on the geographical location of the place.

On average, a general home care facility can cost anything between $1,500 and $4,500 a month. However, homes that provide memory care services may charge $1,000 more. Homes that provide dementia care facilities may cost even more. While some only accept private payments, some personal care services are covered by Medicaid insurance.

A personal care home is one of the best options when it comes to giving a loved one home-like comfort during the later stages of their lives. From a safe living environment to the best nursing facilities, residential home cares offer it all.

Skilled Nursing Facilities - Specialized Medical Services

A Skilled Nursing Home or Facility is a specialized healthcare facility that provides essential medical services to individuals in need. It has one or more registered nurses who provide round-the-clock nursing care. In addition, they have doctors as well as a place to store and distribute medication. Skilled Nursing Facilities (SNFs) handle personal hygiene and daily meals as well. However, there are several federal regulations related to the do's and don'ts of such a nursing facility.

Services Offered by SNF

Apart from basic nursing attention, skilled nursing facilities offer a range of other services to patients. Some of the more common services include but are not limited to speech therapy, occupational therapy, and physical therapy. They also offer other specialized services such as:

- Providing antibiotics and suitable treatment for wounds;

- Helping patients recovering motor skills;

- Providing care for Parkinson's disease (Not all skilled nursing facilities provide this service, be sure to check beforehand);

- Offering services to patients with acute medical conditions, thereby helping them deal with infections, illness, and injuries.

When is the need for SNF?

The need for skilled nursing care is assessed in a hospital or other healthcare institutions. An initial discussion of basic health problems is carried out with patients, along with a clear discharge plan. The commonly stated reasons to consider a skilled nursing facility are as follows:

- Rehabilitation care in case of joint replacements and fractures;
- Acute health conditions;
- Common wound care;
- Diabetic rehabilitation;
- Respiratory care;
- Care for terminal illness;
- Therapy for rapid physical decline and weakness; or
- Need for physical and occupational therapy after stroke or orthopedic procedures such as joint replacement or bone surgery.

How are Payments made for a SNF?

Patients admitted to a SNF usually receive a preliminary health assessment of their mental and physical health. Apart from this, they are subjected to ongoing therapies to evaluate their need for medication and ability to manage daily activities such as decision-making, dressing and bathing.

Some patients need post-hospital care after surgery or acute illness like sepsis. In such cases, many insurance providers cover about 100 days in a nursing facility. Medicare and other insurances usually covers this type of therapy. The admitting person at the skilled nursing home will give us a detailed explanation of that.

A prolonged stay in a nursing facility can prove to be quite expensive. Whatever be the case, most facilities generally have a written record of the expenditure being incurred through the duration of a patient's stay. A copy of this is usually provided to patients for their records.

How is a SNF Different?

The prime factor that sets an SNF apart from other medical institutions is the range and quality of medical services offered. As these facilities specialize in providing round-the-clock services to patients, there are practitioners, nurses and qualified therapists available throughout the day. Professionals at SNFs are skilled at taking care of daily necessities like meals, personal hygiene and daily medication.

Pointers for Choosing a SNF

Elderly people often have the desire to stay within the comfort of their own home. However, this desire needs to be weighed against the essential care that they need, both physically and medically. Here are a few pointers that might help us choose the right SNF:

- Ask about the staff attrition rate at the facility. Ensure that the facility we choose have at least some staff members who have worked there for several years.

- Cleanliness is a prime factor. Strong odors and untidy surroundings can make the stay very uncomfortable and unhygienic. Make sure rooms and other accessories are cleaned regularly.

- Talk to current residents. Find out if they're pleased with the services. Note whether they're wearing clean clothes, are properly groomed and receive quality food.

- Good facilities have dieticians who take care of regular meals offered to patients. Find out about the quality and variety of meals offered.
- Choose a location close to our residence. This makes travelling to the facility easy in case of an emergency.
- Inquire if people responsible for taking care of patients are specialized or experienced in the field of skilled nursing care.

There has been an increase in the popularity of SNFs, given the high-end medical care and convenience they provide. Giving the best of medical attention to our loved ones is no longer a great hassle.

Palliative Care: A Specialized Medical Approach

Palliative care is a specialized medical approach to care for patients suffering from a serious ailment. It is primarily aimed at providing relief from the stress and symptoms of the illness, thereby improving the quality of life. A patient receiving oxygen to ease COPD or severe chronic respiratory failure is receiving palliative care. The treatment is not aimed at curing the disease, it treats the symptoms and improves a patient's quality of life.

Who Can Benefit from It?

Palliative care can be an option for anybody suffering from serious illnesses including chronic lung disease, heart failure, dementia, cancer or neurological disease. Palliative care provides a great deal of relief to the patient and their loved ones. Most importantly, it improves the quality of the patient's life.

This care can also be highly beneficial for the elderly experiencing a great deal of discomfort or frailty in the later stages of life. Since it does not depend much on prognosis, palliative care is often grouped with other remedial forms of treatment. Patients who receive palliative care therapy usually continue other treatments for their illness.

Goals of Palliative Care

- Ease distressing symptoms and pain
- Combines the spiritual and psychological aspects of the patient's care
- Does not aim at either postponing or hastening death

- Enhances the quality of living by positively influencing the duration of the illness
- Acts as a support system helping patients live a healthier and more active life
- Helps families deal with situations related to the person's ailment
- Makes use of a team approach to identify and address the patient's and their family's needs

Who Provides Palliative Care?

Palliative care is generally rendered by palliative care experts and medical practitioners with training and certifications in the field. Such professionals provide all-inclusive care to the patient, concentrating on the emotional, physical, spiritual and social issues faced by the individual and their family during their ailment. These specialists also offer caregiver support and help ease communication within the health-care team.

Palliative care specialists often work as part of a team including nurses, doctors, pharmacists, psychologists, social workers and registered dieticians.

What Does Palliative Care help with?

A serious ailment not only affects the patient's physical well-being, but also other aspects of their life and the lives of the people around them. Palliative care aims to address all these issues.

<u>Social and Emotional Problems</u>

Patients and their families go through an immense amount of stress over the course of a serious illness. Anxiety, fear, depression or a feeling of hopelessness are not uncommon. Palliative care experts help families and individuals deal with these emotions during the diagnostic phase.

Physical Problems

Some common physical effects witnessed during palliative care include:

- Shortness of breath
- Pain
- Troubled sleep
- Lack of appetite or stomach sickness

In all such cases, physicians opt for alternative treatments, nutritional guidance, physical therapy, medicine, integrative therapies or occupational therapies.

Spiritual Issues

Serious health issues may cause patients and their families to doubt their faith. This is most common in patients diagnosed with cancer or other terminal illness. Such patients and their families often struggle to find a deeper meaning of life. A specialized palliative care group helps them explore their values and beliefs, helping them move toward acceptance. They may be able to help us with church services.

Practical Problems

In addition to these issues are the day-to-day practicalities of life such as legal and financial worries, employment issues and insurance questions. Palliative care specialists can help by explaining difficult medical terms or help families pick the right treatment. They may provide financial counselling options to the families and help them find proper housing and transportation resources.

Importance of Communication

Effective communication is an important part of the entire palliative care procedure. A specialized team ensures that they spend enough time talking and listening to the patient, then seeks to form an idea of the patient's personal goals.

They can then incorporate these goals and aspirations into their treatment. Coordination among the doctors is vital, as it helps all involved work for the patent's desired goals.

Consult the physician before and during palliative care. A patient may opt for palliative care at any point of their treatment. Palliative care can be provided at home, hospital or at long-term facility.

Hospice: Caring For the Terminally Ill

Hospice care is provided when curative treatment can no longer help the patient and the expected life span is six months or less. A doctor generally begins the conversation when they think that the patient's prognosis is poor and further medical treatment is futile.

Most people consider hospice care as "the last option" and consider it "giving up." This isn't true. Hospice care is for any patient who has completely stopped responding to treatment of terminal illness. The will to live may remain strong but medical science may have reached its limit. The patient is treated with utmost dignity and receives special care. The goal is to provide maximum comfort to the patient. Hospice care emphasizes on improving the quality of life over the length of life.

A group of able and caring healthcare professionals, nurses, caregivers and volunteers provide the patient with medical assistance, spiritual support and psychological strength during this difficult time. The caregivers try to ease the patient's pain and suffering and make them as comfortable as possible. Many hospice programs also seek to ease the family's suffering as the loss of a loved one appears imminent.

Hospice care can be provided at the patient's home, at a hospital, in a nursing home or in a special inpatient hospice center. The main aspect of hospice care is to be able to provide the patient with a certain quality of life that has dignity, comfort and minimal suffering.

Benefits of Hospice Care

<u>Helps control the symptoms and ease pain</u>

The goal of hospice care is to control pain and keep the symptoms of the illness in check. Considerable effort is put forth to ease the suffering of patients and grant them as much control over their lives as possible. This includes managing pain, nausea, discomfort or other side effects. The hospice team attempts to make the patient feel better so that they can attain peace of mind.

<u>Provides proper home care</u>

When appropriate, hospice care can be provided in the patient's home. If a hospice patient needs to be in a hospital or at inpatient hospice center, the hospice team is involved with the patient's care and provides the ambience and comfort like home.

<u>Spiritual support</u>

Since the religious and spiritual needs and beliefs of people differ, the hospice team ensures the patient's needs are met.

<u>Provides healthy interaction</u>

Hospice nurses or social workers regularly meet with the patient and their loved ones. The patient's condition is explained and everyone gets a chance to discuss their feelings and learn about the process of dying. The meetings help provide emotional support to the patient and their families.

<u>Reliability</u>

Hospice teams are generally active 24/7. They have strong team communication which ensures the passing of vital information to everyone from doctors to volunteers. The patients and their families are encouraged to contact the hospice team at any time of the day, in case of any problem or emergency. They are always there to help, which provides a sense of security.

Relieves stress for family members

Since some patients are taken care of at home, it can restrict the activities of family members. This is where hospice services can help. Hospice caregivers can free up time for the patient's near and dear ones, who may dearly need it as caregiving is stressful and can take a toll on one's health. So, respite care can be arranged for up to five days where the patient is taken care of in a hospice facility or in an inpatient setting.

Bereavement support

The hospice care team supports and extends a hand toward the patient's family members and loved ones after the patient's death. During the mourning period, a professional counselor or clergy member is assigned to provide support through visits, phone calls or support groups. The death of a loved one can cause an emotional upheaval. The hospice care team cares about those who are left behind and provides them with assistance and support for about a year after the patient passes away.

How does it begin?

Hospice care may begin as soon as the doctor sends a formal referral to a hospice care service. The representative from the hospice should visit the patient within 48 hours. Following that, the physician will be consulted and a meeting will be held with the patient and their family. All of this will be done after a schedule is arranged, keeping in mind the comfort of the patient and their primary caregiver.

Hospice care begins immediately, within a day or two after the referral is made, depending on the case. Hospice services can be requested by a patient or their family. A formal evaluation to check the eligibility of the patient to receive hospice care will then be scheduled.

How do we choose the right hospice?

The most efficient way to find a suitable hospice is to consult our local hospice provider and discuss their services and whether they'll be suitable for our situation. As the needs of each patient are specific, consulting various hospice providers at the outset is a must. We need to know if they will be able to meet the patient's specific needs and create a suitable environment for them.

Choosing hospice care is an important decision for a patient suffering from a life-limiting illness. Therefore, it needs to be done judiciously.

Hospice care gives both the patient and their family the much-needed support for a better quality of life.

<u>Incurable illness</u>

When dealing with illness, the terms "cure" and "treatment" are easily confused and sometimes are used interchangeably. But they have very different meanings. "Cure" means the condition has been eradicated. It is gone. Some conditions cannot be cured -- the situation is managed through treatment. An infection can be cured but osteoarthritis cannot be cured.

Some of the incurable diseases found in elderly people include:

- Certain types of Cancers
- Heart diseases
- Cerebrovascular disease
- Osteoporosis
- Neuro degenerative diseases

When a person is diagnosed with one of these incurable conditions it affects the entire family. To successfully deal with the disease, family members need to be able to talk about it. When a person learns they have an incurable illness, they're likely to go through a host of emotions - fear, anger and depression are the most likely. Lending a sympathetic ear can go a long way to making a frightening process more bearable.

Talking about illness

Here are some tips for talking with a loved one about their diagnosis:

1. Offer them the opportunity to talk about it, but don't push things. People process in different ways -- and on different timelines. We may be ready and willing to talk but our loved one may not. If not, make sure he or she knows we are ready to listen when they're ready to talk.

2. Don't lead the conversation, our role is to listen. Let our loved one vent. Listen to his or her fears and be patient if they become angry. They are probably angry at the situation, even if it seems they are lashing out at us.

3. Don't judge, don't denigrate. Don't say, "You have nothing to worry about," or "It's silly to be scared." Dismissing their emotions, even if we are trying to reassure them, will make our loved one less likely to open up to us in the future. They may internalize and brood over their fears and anger, which can be harmful to their mental and emotional state.

4. If we and our loved one focus on the incurability of the disease, it is easy to feel discouraged and lose hope of any possible improvement. Focus on what can be done to control the situation and make their life as normal as possible.

5. Seek out a support group - for both our loved one and us. Many people diagnosed with an incurable disease find it more comfortable to talk and connect with people with a similar problem. Sharing our fears, pain, insecurities, and thoughts with other patients helps them reconnect to the society and can improve mental and emotional health.

Living with illness

Some incurable conditions are terminal, others are not. Regardless of our loved one's prognosis, here are some general guidelines to help with living with their condition.

1. Try to live as normally as possible. Go for movie nights, take picnics and plan family dinner as we used to do before their diagnosis. Illness is a complication to be dealt with not a barrier to daily activity.

2. Talk regularly. Arrange a weekly or monthly session to talk about the ups and downs they're experiencing. Both us and our loved one will likely find comfort in the routine of sharing.

3. Laugh, and make them laugh, As the saying goes, laughter is the best medicine. Humor lifts the spirit and is good for emotional health. Read them funny books and funny stories, tell them about something that happened at work or college.

4. Don't encourage false hopes. Be realistic about their prognosis. If the condition is terminal, pretending that death is not coming will only make things more difficult in the long run.

5. Create a bucket list and help them fulfill some of their dreams. The last stage of dying is a depressing time. When it comes, it will make things easier if our loved one can look back on good memories rather than a lifetime of regrets and missed opportunities.

Part I

Mental conditions of the elderly loved ones

Depression

Mary first came to my office as a new patient after her 70th birthday. She looked sad and a little disheveled. She had a history of mild breathing issues and heart problems. She had been to the ER and to my office multiple times for fatigue and weakness. She was seen and cleared by both a pulmonologist and cardiologist. Multiple investigative tests found no issues.

She said she cries often and can't sleep. She said she stays in bed a lot and complains of shortness of breath on mild exertion. She was offered psychotherapy and some depression pills. She was told to follow up after six weeks. At that follow-up, she was a different person. She was smiling, made eye contact, reported sleeping well and had more energy. At three months' follow-up, she had reverted into her normal previous self and has resumed her golf and bridge with friends.

What is depression?

The Oxford dictionary defines depression as feelings of severe despondency and dejection. However, there are various considerations that may conflate the diagnosis of depression. Let us consider how depression differs among the elderly; diagnostic criteria, symptoms, causes and the wide-spanning consequences.

Currently, depression in the elderly is underdiagnosed and undertreated*. While more than six million American above age 65 have depression, only 10 percent receive treatment for it. It is imperative for us to address depression in this population because it can significantly lower their quality of life.

Depression DSM-5 Diagnostic Criteria

The DSM-5 (the official diagnostic and statistical manual for mental disorders) outlines the following criteria to make a diagnosis of depression. The individual must be experiencing five or more symptoms during the same two-week period and at least one of the symptoms should be either (1) depressed mood or (2) loss of interest or pleasure.

1. Depressed mood most of the day, nearly every day.

2. Markedly diminished interest or pleasure in all, or almost all, activities most of the day, nearly every day.

3. Significant weight loss when not dieting or weight gain, or decrease or increase in appetite nearly every day.

4. A slowing down of thought and a reduction of physical movement (observable by others, not merely subjective feelings of restlessness or being slowed down).

5. Fatigue or loss of energy nearly every day.

6. Feelings of worthlessness or excessive or inappropriate guilt nearly every day.

7. Diminished ability to think or concentrate, or indecisiveness, nearly every day.

8. Recurrent thoughts of death, recurrent suicidal ideation without a specific plan, or a suicide attempt or a specific plan for committing suicide.

While these criteria are similar for all individuals, depression in older adults is often misinterpreted. It is important for the elderly and their loved ones to remain careful because senile depression can be difficult to identify. Often times, the symptoms of depression can be confused with stress or a normal part of aging. It is also possible for it to be dismissed as a side effect of medicine. Because so-called "mild depression" is prevalent amongst older adults, families often pay little attention to these feelings. Family members and even many doctors will be focused on the physical health component of aging to a point that they will completely ignore the symptoms and signs of depression.

In order to effectively combat missing these important diagnoses, it is important for us to know what a depression symptom look like. Here are some of the most common symptoms to watch out for in our parent or person we are caring for:

a) Tired all the time

b) Not sleeping well

c) Lack of energy

d) Poor appetite

e) Weight loss

f) Pain all over

g) Belly pain all the time, with normal test results

h) Forgetful (Not all forgetfulness is dementia)

i) Unhappy

j) Not as organized as she/he used to be

k) Unkempt

l) Sad since some close friend or family member passed away

m) Not able to concentrate well

n) Afraid that she/he may die soon

Any of these symptoms alone are not cause for concern, but if an elderly loved one begins exhibiting multiple symptoms on this list a discussion with him or her (or their doctor) should be considered.

Causes of depression in older adults:

It frequently is difficult to identify the source of depression due to the wide range of social and cultural influences that may affect our loved ones. Depression symptoms may randomly appear out of nowhere one day. In these cases, it is also possible that our elderly loved one was attempting to hide their feelings and pain. It is also possible for the depression symptoms to appear after a significant change in life, such as losing independency to the death of a loved one to financial challenges.

Research has shown that depression is more likely in certain demographics:

- Women have more chance of depression than men.
- Single people have more depression than those who are married.
- Socially isolated people are more prone to depression than those who are socially-connected with friends and family.
- Elderly loved ones with prior history of psychiatric disorders will have greater chances of developing depression due to life changing events.
- Patients with these medical conditions are more likely to have depression:
  - heart failure
  - atrial fibrillation
  - recent falls
  - recent major surgeries

- chronic lung problems
- arthritis
- neurological disorders like multiple sclerosis or Parkinson's
- cancer

What are the consequences of untreated depression in older persons?

Untreated depression significantly lowers the quality of life for our loved one. Complications of depression prevent elderly loved ones from enjoying life around them and it can make them feel as though life is not worth living.

Suicide rates amongst older adults is quite high. According to the American Association for Marriage and Family Therapy (AAMFT), those 85 or older have the highest rate of suicide in America. The second and third highest age groups are 75- to 85-year-olds and 65- to 75-year-olds, respectively. All suicides cannot be attributed to depression but depression can lead to suicides.

Diagnosing depression among the elderly

If we think that our loved one may be suffering from depression, then talk to a primary care doctor (preferably a geriatrician) or a psychiatrist. They will help assess our situation and make a proper diagnosis. It is important to discuss the situation with a trained professional rather than trying to research the issue ourself on the internet. Many issues may exhibit identical symptoms and only through face to face discussion can a trained professional make an accurate diagnosis.

Treating depression among the elderly

After gathering a detailed history of the patient, the doctor may order further tests to rule out other illnesses. If the diagnosis is depression, the doctor may prescribe medications to address the symptoms. Doctors may prescribe a sedative to help with sleeping issues, or possibly an antidepressant. The manner of treatment will depend on the patient's condition and the doctor's preference. Drugs referred to as SSRIs and SNRIs are the top classes of medications prescribed for depression and usually take six to eight weeks to work effectively.

A patient also may be sent for psychotherapy. Psychotherapy, or talk therapy, helps people with numerous mental illnesses and emotional problems. It is also helpful for people going through major stresses in life, such as a diagnosis of cancer or loss of loved ones.

Older adults may have a tough time accepting a diagnosis of depression. Even though depression is a well-known illness, there used to be a lot of stigma attached to psychiatric problems and some of that still lingers, especially with older generations.

How depression affects the family and close friends and what can we do about it?

Psychiatric illnesses not only affect the elderly loved one, but also the family and close friends. They become sad when they see their loved one going through a tough time. As a family:

- We need to be around our elderly loved ones.
- We need to make sure that their needs are met.
- We need to make sure that they don't feel lonely.

- We need to take them to church or shopping or to the park for a leisurely stroll.
- We need to make sure that they take the meds properly
- We need to make sure that they are keeping their appointment with the doctors.
- We need to involve them in new activities or the activities they love.
- We need to help them find depression support groups
- We need to help them find volunteering opportunities

By working together to help our elderly loved one find a purpose in life and help them cope with their challenges, we will drastically improve their quality of life.

Anxiety

A 76-year-old patient came to my office. When he stood up, he started shaking and swaying sideways, as if he was falling. However, he had no history of falls. He and his wife care for his ailing 95-year-old mother-in-law. His symptoms have been going on for three months and in general has been more worried in his day-to-day life. He has seen a couple of doctors in the past and CT scans of his head were normal. I sent him for psychotherapy and started him on a low dose of SSRI. In two months, his symptoms resolved completely.

Anxiety disorder is an emotional experience in which a person experiences discomfort from the uncertainty of perspective; the mind is not able to relax. A person with an anxiety disorder is in a state of nervousness most of the time and can do nothing about it. The Geriatric Mental Health Foundation furthers the definition by stating "feelings of fear, worry, apprehension, or dread that are excessive or disproportionate to the problems or situations that are feared."

One in four adult Americans will have at least one episode of an anxiety disorder in their lifetime. Additionally, up to 15% of elderly Americans suffer from some type of anxiety disorder. Studies show most anxiety disorders in the elderly are chronic and usually occur earlier in life, except for Generalized Anxiety Disorder (GAD) and Agoraphobia, which may turn up later in life. However, late-life GAD is largely undetected and untreated in primary care.

Anxiety can be associated with depression, even when depression is not necessarily a prominent feature. Anxiety is also related with hypochondria -- fear of a disease that isn't present or fear that a minor illness is much more severe.

The presentation of an anxiety disorder varies a lot. Here are some of the typical presenting features:

1. Chest pain all the time and the heart doctor has ruled out any type of heart diseases
2. Feeling of heart racing off and on (Panic attack, but heart problems need to be ruled out)
3. Complains of shortness of breath at times
4. Visits bathroom frequently (urinary causes need to be ruled out)
5. Has terrible fear of death
6. Symptoms of nausea and lightheadedness.
7. Wants to take a shower 3 to 4 times a day (obsessive compulsive)
8. Mops the kitchen all the time (obsessive compulsive)
9. Experiences a childhood assault and has nightmares (PTSD)
10. Is more irritable than usual
11. Gets distracted easily
12. Wants to stay at home all the time and gets nervous in church or at parties (Social anxiety)
13. Used to be adventurous/travel but now is even scared of flying
14. Worries about every small thing which happens around her

Who is at risk?

While no one is exempt from the possibility of having an anxiety disorder, some older adults are more likely than others. Risk factors may include:

1. Chronic lung diseases, such as emphysema
2. Heart problems
3. Physical limitations because of debilitating arthritis or a stroke
4. Medications like steroids and inhalers
5. Poverty
6. Stressful life events
7. Alcohol, drug or prescription drug abuse

Other aggravating factors include:

1. Women develop anxiety disorder twice as often as men.
2. Having an immediate relative suffering an anxiety disorder.
3. Having been raised under conditions of excessive care or who had experience of early ill-treatment, are also at risk.
4. Having experienced extreme stress, trauma, bereavement or chronic grief
5. Having alcohol or drug problems
6. Having a family history of anxiety disorders
7. Having other medical, mental illnesses or dementia.

Our elderly loved ones need to avoid things that can aggravate the symptoms of anxiety disorders such as:

- Caffeine
- Nicotine
- Overeating
- Over-the-counter cold medications

- Certain illegal drugs
- Some herbal supplements e.g. ginseng
- Alcohol*

*While alcohol might initially help a person relax, it eventually interferes with sleep and overall wellness and can even contribute to anxiety, depression and dementia.

Consequences of untreated anxiety disorder

Untreated anxiety can spill over into multiple areas of life.

1. Anxiety disorder is likely to become chronic, with the victim suffering for the rest of his or her life.
2. There is a considerable risk that anxiety sufferers will also develop depression.
3. Anxiety can lead to trouble remembering, learning new things, concentrating or decision-making.
4. Anxiety can lead to disability, poor physical health and a poor quality of life.

An older adult suffering from anxiety disorder may live in a constant state of alarm or tension. This will not only affect his or her day-to-day activities but will also impact his or her sleep. This will lead to chronic fatigue, which significantly lowers quality of life.

Late-life Generalized Anxiety Disorder also has been linked to increased risk of stroke and other cardiovascular events as well as an increased risk of mild cognitive impairment advancing into Alzheimer's disease.

This constant state of anxiety can damage relationships with family and friends as well. Having to listen to a constant litany of fears or impending misfortune - especially when the anxiety sufferer cannot be convinced that all is well - may drive a wedge between the patient and those who care about him or her. This, in turn, can lead to increased isolation and increased anxiety.

Individuals with pathologically high anxiety demonstrate worse day-to-day planning skills, inefficiently cope with routine tasks, and tend to postpone important issues, which worsens their anxiety. Anxiety disorders will rarely improve without deliberate effort and likely will worsen.

Anxiety treatment in Older Adults

As with depression, diagnosis and treatment of anxiety begins with a conversation with a doctor, who will seek a detailed history of the patient's mental state and how it may have devolved into anxiety. There may be tests to rule out other conditions before a diagnosis of anxiety.

Treatment of anxiety disorders involves:

1. Cognitive behavioral therapy;
2. SSRI (Selective serotonin reuptake inhibitors); and
3. Benzodiazepines and other medication in severe cases.

According to The American Association of Geriatric Psychiatry, "cognitive behavioral therapy, or psychotherapy, involves talking with a trained mental health professional, such as a psychiatrist, psychologist, social worker, or counselor, to discover what caused the anxiety disorder and how to deal with its symptoms. In cognitive-behavioral therapy, therapists help people change the thinking patterns that contribute to their fears and the ways they react to anxiety-provoking situations.

A therapist can teach new coping and relaxation skills and help resolve problems that cause anxiety. When a patient is ready to face his or her fears, a therapist can teach exposure techniques to desensitize the patient to the situations that trigger anxious feelings. Therapists also teach deep breathing and other relaxation techniques to relieve anxiety. Behavioral therapy is short-term therapy of twelve or fewer sessions."

SSRIs such as Prozac, Zoloft and Lexapro etc. are among a selection of medications that, in conjunction with psychotherapy, are key in anxiety treatment. It is important to remember that while these drugs help individuals cope with worries and nervousness, they can take from four to eight weeks to generate a result. SSRIs also have fewer side effects than older generation antidepressants.

Buspirone can also be used in elderly loved ones for anxiety. As far as benzodiazepines are concerned, they are used very often. However, use of benzodiazepines like Xanax and Valium is associated with more drowsiness, confusion, and falls. Therefore, it is better to avoid benzodiazepines as much as possible.

How Can We Help?

As with any psychiatric disorder, anxiety affects the whole family. It can be heartbreaking to see a loved one under the constant anxiety-produced stress. But as the disease lingers, it is also normal to become desensitized to the stress and consider it a side effect of aging.

But with the right course of medical treatment and a little patience and understanding, we can help a loved one overcome their affliction.

Here are some tips for helping an elderly loved one struggling with anxiety:

- Be around in their tough time.
- Be calm and reassuring.
- Make sure their physical and psychological needs are met.

- Make sure that they don't feel lonely.
- Acknowledge their fears but avoid supporting the fear.
- Take them out -- go to church, go shopping or take a leisurely stroll in the park.
- Make sure they take their medication.
- Make sure they are going to their appointments with the doctors.
- Involve them in new activities or restart an old one that they love.
- Encourage them to engage in social activities.
- Help them find volunteering opportunities.
- Help them with financial planning and finances if possible.
- Help them adopt stress management techniques like meditation, prayer, chanting or deep breathing.
- Limit their access to news of current events. Too much negative news can contribute to anxiety.

By working together to help our elderly loved one find a sense of purpose in life and help them cope with their challenges, we will drastically improve their quality of life.

Dementia

Dementia is a degenerative brain illness which affects a person's memory, reasoning, judgement, insight and other cognitive abilities. It causes a decline in mental and physical functioning, which leads to slow deterioration of language, communication and calculation skills and it even can affect mobility.

According to the World Health Organization (WHO), about 50 million people worldwide suffer with dementia. A new case is diagnosed every three seconds. WHO estimates about 7 percent of people 65 or older have dementia, with slightly higher rates (8 to 10 percent) in developed countries due to longer life spans.

Dementia isn't just one simple disease —it acts like a host of diseases. And different types of dementia have different prognoses and different life expectancies. Major risk factors of dementia include advancing age, genetic profile and systemic vascular disease.

There are multiple types of dementia. Here are some of the biggest categories:

1) Alzheimer's disease

Alzheimer's disease is the most common neurodegenerative dementia. It can strike any middle-aged or older adult.

Alzheimer's disease has a prevalence of 5-6% of all individuals age 65 and above. This percent rises up to 30% for those over age 85. About 5% of all Alzheimer's disease occurs before age 65, which is conventionally termed "early-onset".

The disease typically begins with slow, progressive memory decline. Behavioral, visuospatial or language dysfunction dominate in less common variants.

The life expectancy in an Alzheimer's patient is around ten years, although this can vary depending on the patient's age and overall general health.

To date, there are no disease-modifying, pharmacologic treatments for Alzheimer's disease. Research has focused on early detection and therapeutic targeting of the tissues altered by the disease.17 Current medications do not alter the overall course of decline, but they may improve cognitive and behavioral symptoms for periods of six months to several years. 18,19. They are usually recommended for a year or so. I have noticed that stopping these medicines can cause adverse effects, so if a doctor recommends discontinuing them, it might be wise to taper off slowly before stopping.

Evidence suggests that regular aerobic exercise, adherence to a Mediterranean-style diet and participation in socially and cognitively stimulating activities can decrease one's risk of Alzheimer's disease and possibly slow its progression. 20,21

2) Dementia with Lewy bodies, Parkinson's disease, and multiple system atrophy.

Dementia with Lewy bodies (LBD) is probably the second most common degenerative dementia after Alzheimer's. According to the Lewy body association, the average life expectancy is five to seven years, but can be as long as 20 years.

We may observe these

- Mom is unable to plan or process the information.
- Mom has a lot of hallucinations, she is seeing things which are not there.
- Mom is acting out her dreams.
- Mom's attention span and alertness has decreased, she has developed ADD.
- Mom passes urine on herself without realising.
- Mom has tremors in the hands, is stiff and walks slowly.
- Mom is not as alert as she used to be.

These motor, cognitive and sleep symptoms can also be features of the dementia associated with Parkinson's disease. Conventionally, Parkinson's disease dementia should be used to describe dementia that develops in the setting of well-established Parkinson disease, and should occur at least one year after the onset of parkinsonism.

Many traditional antipsychotic medications (for example, Haloperidol, Risperdal, Quetiapine) are sometimes prescribed for individuals with Alzheimer's disease and other forms of dementia to control behavioral symptoms. However, LBD and Parkinson's disease dementia affects an individual's brain differently than other dementias. As a result, these medications can cause a severe worsening of movement and a potentially fatal condition known as neuroleptic malignant syndrome (NMS). NMS causes severe fever, muscle rigidity and breakdown that can lead to kidney failure.

3) The frontotemporal dementia

Frontotemporal dementias are probably the third most common type of degenerative dementia. In patients younger than 65, frontotemporal dementias are the second most common dementia after Alzheimer's disease, accounting for close to 20 percent of all cases.

In this dementia, behavioral and language problems will be more prominent initially, than the memory loss. We may observe these symptoms and behaviors in our loved ones:

- difficulty in reading, writing and even understanding certain words
- trouble recalling the name of everyday objects like spoon, knife, pen etc. This is called anomia
- non-fluent speech. She makes grammatical mistakes while talking
- doesn't care about her personal hygiene anymore
- has started to eat "everything" for a few days. Over eating.
- lost interest in her hobbies and work at home. (Apathy)
- makes offensive and rude comments about other people. (Disinhibition)
- makes obscene hand gestures to strangers. (Disinhibition)
- was caught stealing from Walmart. (Disinhibition)
- someone died but it didn't faze her at all; no emotions shown by her. (Emotional blunting)
- reading the same book again and again. (Compulsive behavior)

How Can We Help?

This is one of the nastiest dementias of all. The patient's family and friends must be patient and empathetic. The patient may need to be moved to a skilled facility earlier than with other forms of dementia to deal with behavioral issues. Elderly loved one may need frequent visits to a primary care doctor as well as psychiatrist.

Medical treatment for the frontotemporal dementias is supportive, with a focus on relieving neuropsychiatric and motor symptoms with antidepressants and dopamine-modulating therapy, respectively; response to dopaminergic medications is usually poor.

4) Vascular dementia

Diseases such as Alzheimers, Lewy body and frontotemporal are all degenerative — cells of the nervous system degenerate or stop working. Vascular dementia, on the other hand, is characterized by having problems in providing ample blood supply to the brain, leading to worsening cognitive decline. It is generally caused by a stroke or multiple strokes or small vessel ischemic disease. Vascular dementia accounts for about 15 to 35 percent of all dementia diagnoses.

Individuals with vascular dementia are prone to strokes and heart diseases, which leads to shorter life spans. The average lifespan of a patient diagnosed with vascular dementia is about four years, although early detection and treatment can extend the life expectancy.

Patients with vascular dementia are treated the same as stroke patients. The patient is prescribed a statin to control cholesterol, blood pressure and blood sugar are regulated (usually through the use of medications) and the patient may be prescribed low-dose aspirin or other blood thinning medicines.

Evaluation of dementia

The initial evaluation and diagnosis of dementia should include at least the following four elements:

1. A thorough clinical history;
2. A neurological exam, with an emphasis on the assessment of mental status. Tests such as the Mini Mental State Examination (MMSE) and the Montreal Cognitive Assessment (MoCA) have good sensitivity and specificity. However, neither assess for problems with mood or thought content. Both altered mood and abnormal thought content can have a strong impact on cognitive function. Therefore, all the patients with signs of dementia should be screened for depression as well, because depression can have negative effects on memory and cognition;
3. Selective labs to screen for selected metabolic/physiologic abnormalities (e.g., basic chemistries, complete blood count, thyroid panel, B12, Vitamin D).
4. A structural brain scan, with MRI preferable to CT whenever possible. MRI and CT scans are not done always. Usually, they are done in patients with fast decline in mental and physical condition. Many people with symptoms of frontotemporal dementia should get scans for appropriate diagnosis. Again, it will be at the doctor's discretion to order them according to patient's condition.

Stages of Dementia

There are several methods that are widely used to predict the stages of dementia, however the most widely practiced scale is the Global Deterioration Scale (GDS), commonly known as Reisberg Scale. GDS is usually used for staging of Alzheimer's dementia.

For simplicity, we will categorize all types dementia into three stages: mild, moderate, and severe. Our goal is to understand the tough decisions associated with dementia.

Mild cognitive impairment (MCI)

Mild cognitive impairment causes cognitive changes that are noticeable to the patient or people who regularly interact with them. These changes, however, do not affect daily life or the dementia patient's autonomous function.

This is the stage between the expected cognitive decline of normal aging and the more serious decline of dementia. It can involve problems with memory, language, thinking and judgment that are greater than normal age-related changes.

People with MCI, especially MCI including memory problems, are more likely to develop Alzheimer's or other dementia than individuals without MCI. However, MCI does not necessarily lead to further dementia. In a few people, the MCI remains stable or even disappears.

MCI can develop as a side effect of medication, so it's critical that people experiencing cognitive impairment seek help as soon as possible. Family and friends have to be more vigilant at this stage as these symptoms can be tied to hypothyroidism, depression, occult cancers or vitamin B12 deficiency.

Make sure that loved ones are evaluated by a good physician who is well versed in managing those symptoms. This is a good time to open discussions about financial issues, living wills and trusts. Other issues that should be addressed include advanced care directives and planning with our elderly loved ones. Onset of MCI should spur a person to act to ensure that issues, people and items close to their heart are addressed.

Mild Dementia

Mild Dementia patients do have forgetfulness but still function independently. They may have some depression type symptoms. They . Start having financial management problem, start misplacing things, start calculation problems. Some patients don't acknowledge that they have any memory issues. They will need to see the dementia specialist and if the tests confirm mild dementia then patients can take medicines to improve the symptoms to some degree.

Moderate Dementia

Patient suffering from moderate dementia may exhibit these symptoms:

- Decreased performance at work
- Increased episodes of memory loss
- Trouble understanding complex instructions
- Stuttering and/or difficulty in conversations and speech
- Misplacing personal belongings
- Difficulty in recalling fresh memories or recent conversations
- Cutting off of friends or family
- Increase in the severity of mental illness such as anxiety, depression and irritability
- Trouble remembering names and routes and trouble driving
- Inability to plan and organize events and activities
- Skipping meals
- Trouble travelling or trouble living alone

Usually during this situation, the elderly person is isolated as their caregiver or loved ones are unable to understand and fulfill their need for interaction and stimulation. Murna Downs, a professor of dementia at the University of Bradford, once said "you cannot put a child on a chair and make him stay there all day doing nothing. Just like that child, loved ones with dementia need human contact and stimulation'.

Moderate dementia makes caring for our loved ones more of a challenge for the caregiver, as the person's behavior changes, bringing frequent episodes of rage and memory loss.

We need to provide more care and attention to our loved ones during this stage. When a person is suffering from moderate dementia, family and friends will have to make an intervention in their life - the sufferer has physical and emotional needs that they can no longer deal with on their own.

This is the stage where most of the critical decision-making needs to be done. We likely will have to make at least one tough decision, such as whether the person can safely live alone or whether they need some form of assistance. Other issues that may need to be addressed are whether it is still safe for our loved one to drive or own firearms.

Here is a list of questions to consider:

- Can our loved one be cared for appropriately at home?
- Does our loved one need adult day care service help?
- Does our loved one need 24/7 care at home?
- Will our loved one be safe at home?
- Does our loved one have access to three meals a day?
- Can we or our loved one afford the care which can be provided at home?
- Does our loved one have long term care insurance?

- Does our loved one need to be in assisted living place or in skilled nursing?
- Should our loved one have access to firearms?
- Should our loved one need to be driving? Are they putting their life or the life of others in danger by driving? Are they safe on the road?

So here are the things to look for. Checking the following boxes can easily help us find the right care for our loved ones:

- [ ] Wandering
- [ ] Driving problems
- [ ] Falls
- [ ] Leaving the door open at night
- [ ] Leaving the stove burning
- [ ] Other safety problems
- [ ] Need of 24/7 care at home
- [ ] Help needed at night
- [ ] Help need in the day time
- [ ] Don't remember anything
- [ ] Bed bound
- [ ] Not eating
- [ ] Not able to swallow
- [ ] Losing weight
- [ ] Does our loved one know our name
- [ ] Spouse and kids can't take care

Severe Dementia:

A patient with severe dementia has many of these symptoms

- Finding it hard to eat and swallow food
- Not recognizing anyone
- No bowel or bladder control
- Severe changes in the weight of the person, typically weight loss
- The gradual loss of speaking ability
- Restlessness and anxiety
- Hallucinations and delusions
- Angry outbursts and episodes of rage due to confusion
- Weakened immune system leaving a loved one vulnerable to infections like pneumonia
- Limited mobility, or an inability to walk or stand up
- Becoming bed bound or wheelchair bound
- Not taking medicine

During very severe cognitive decline, we may have to consider palliative care or hospice to fulfill the physical, mental, and emotional needs of our elderly loved one and ensure their comfort. It is a time when we will have to start making decisions about dignity and quality of life.

While a feeding tube may be needed to prolong a loved one's life, this is the stage where we may have to confront the fact that extending a loved one's life might not be the best decision. A loved one who is not eating may not be doing so because their body is shutting down.

This is the time to talk openly and honestly with doctors about a prognosis. Does the doctor think that our loved one has six months left to live? No doctor can give us a definite answer but doctors who care for dementia patients will have a rough idea.

The conversation may be heart-wrenching, but it is also necessary. Here are some questions and topics to discuss at this stage of a patient's life:

- How much longer do we think our loved one will live? Are we talking years, months or just weeks?
- Do we think that the medicines are no longer necessary? Remember to reduce the burden of unnecessary pills in elderly loved ones.
- Does my loved one need palliative care?
- Does my loved one need hospice care?

During the last few days of dementia, the prevailing conditions worsen. Due to decreased blood flow and bodily activity, our loved one might have cold hands and arms. He or she may stop eating or swallowing any food or water. They might become more agitated or restless. During the last stage our loved ones may have trouble breathing normally. Their agitation may lead to screaming, moaning, restlessness or sweating.

Dementia is an ugly brain disease that takes a toll on all involved.

While caring for a loved one, family and friends must care for themselves as well. It is a stressful time and we need to be at our best to provide our best to others.

PART II

HEALTH OF THE ELDERLY LOVED ONES

Heart Disease

Heart disease is the number one cause of death in elderly. With age we develop a condition called atherosclerosis, which is stiffness of the blood vessels. This condition can cause myocardial infarction or what is commonly known as heart attack. Some people don't have a heart attack, but they have chest pain due to atherosclerosis and it is called angina. These types of patients need to see the doctor immediately for evaluation.

According to the American College of Cardiology, high blood pressure remains the number one heart condition in people above age 75. Other heart conditions include coronary artery disease, congestive heart failure, irregular heartbeat and a condition called atrial fibrillation.

When to consult a Doctor?

If an elderly loved one suffer symptoms such as shortening of breath, progressive fatigue, chest pain, variable heartbeat, frequent changes in blood pressure or dizziness, SEE A DOCTOR IMMEDIATELY. All these symptoms can indicate heart disease.

Problems of the Heart:

<u>Angina pectoris</u> is pain in the left side of the chest; it also might be experienced as tightness in the chest. It can be caused by emotional and physical distress and is common in older people. Angina pectoris without pain, also known as silent ischemia, also can be common among the elderly.

<u>Acute Coronary Syndrome</u> A heart attack, or symptoms that warn one may be imminent, can be classified as ACS. This syndrome becomes

more frequent and intense as we age. An electrocardiogram (ECG) is a simple diagnostic tool used to detect Acute Coronary Syndrome.

In seniors ACS may go unnoticed, unless the loved ones and caregivers have noticed shortness of breath, sudden fatigue and restlessness.

<u>Chronic Heart Failure</u> When the heart is unable to pump enough blood, it is called heart failure. The muscles of the heart may have weakened or may be unable to relax. Common signs of heart failure include fatigue, shortness of breath, swollen legs and restlessness. As with ACS, the chance of heart failure increases with age. Even if well treated and given proper medication heart failure leads to more frequent death in older people than in young individuals.

<u>Irregular, too slow or too fast heartbeat</u> Patients might feel palpitations in their chest. Some other signs of this problem include sweating, pallor, weakness, occasional dizziness and syncope -- passing out.

A slow heartbeat is a direct consequence of problems with the electrical system in the heart. To tackle the issue, a sophisticated heart device known as a pacemaker is sometimes implanted in the patient's chest to maintain a normal heartbeat.

Preventive Measures

Although aging itself brings a significant risk for cardiovascular dysfunction, there are some things we can do to help prevent heart disease.

- Avoid smoking (both passive and active smoking are hazardous)
- Make exercise and physical activity part of a daily routine.
- Control blood pressure by maintaining a balanced diet. (avoid oily food and make fruits and vegetables a significant portion of the daily diet)

- Maintain regular eating and sleeping patterns.
- Use medication or a balanced diet to control cholesterol levels.

Here are some points to consider while taking care of a loved one with a heart condition:

1. Is the chest pain debilitating?
2. Is the shortness of breath debilitating?
3. Can the patient lay flat? (A need for additional pillows can be a sign of heart failure)
4. Is the loved one able to take care of him- or herself?
5. Is the loved one taking medicines properly?
6. Is the medication affordable?
7. Do doctors recommend more procedures?
8. What is the life expectancy? (Speak with the doctors)
9. In case of heart failure ask the cardiologist how bad is the heart failure? What type of heart failure it is? is it weakness of the muscle or is it stiffness of the muscle of the heart?
10. On the scale of 1 to 10, what does the patient think, how bad is their condition?
11. On the scale of 1 to 10, what do we think about the patient's condition? Are they able to take care of themselves?
12. Does our loved one need occasional help or help through the whole day?
13. Does our loved one need help at night or in the day time?

14. Does our loved one need help with groceries and shopping?

Considering these questions will help family and friends determine whether an elderly loved one can stay in their home alone or with assistance or whether they need to move to a personal care home or assisted living facility.

Lung Conditions

According to the Centers for Disease Control and Prevention (CDC), one in seven elderly people suffer some kind of pulmonary (lung) problem. These include asthma and Chronic Obstructive Pulmonary Disease (COPD), such as emphysema or chronic bronchitis.

Many of these patients have a cough and shortness of breath. In many patients, the problem may be severe enough to require oxygen therapy and greatly affect the patient's quality of life.

Asthma is a common problem in older people which is usually neglected and considered as a common symptom of aging. While asthma itself is manageable, it can create obstacles in the treatment and diagnosis of other diseases.

According to Asthma and Allergy Foundation of America (AAFA), older asthma patients require more medication than younger ones and may need someone to monitor them to ensure all is well as mild asthma can escalate into a respiratory failure without warning.

Progressive lung diseases such as chronic bronchitis or emphysema are generally referred to as Chronic Obstructive Pulmonary Disease (COPD). The two major causes of COPD are smoking (or passive smoke) and aging. As per COPD foundation, COPD is the fourth most common cause of death in the United States.

Other lung-related diseases include pulmonary fibrosis, respiratory distress syndrome and sarcoidosis as well as upper airway conditions such as chronic sinusitis and rhinitis.

As we age, our bones may become thinner. This loss of bone density may allow the ribcage to change shape and become more rigid, making breathing more difficult. This may lead to anger or depression and cause the sufferer to lash out at family and friends. Or they may isolate themselves.

Older people are more prone to respiratory infections such as bronchitis or pneumonia, both of which feature coughing, fever and mucus. A patient may face difficulty in eating and swallowing, as his or her airways become infected or swollen, squeezing the esophagus.

Someone with lung diseases might have normal breathing and heart rate when at rest, but cannot take part in physical activity as he or she becomes short of breath while doing that particular activity

When we observe our loved one facing difficulty in breathing, we should immediately consult a doctor. The condition is even worse in a dementia patient as they may not be able to articulate the history properly.

The role of caregiver in case of chronic lung diseases

- If our elderly loved one has asthma or COPD, we can help them by working to eliminate cigarettes, smoke, dust, pollen, animal dander and perfume from their environment.
- Make sure they take medication on time. If they have a prescribed inhaler, ensure it is with them at all times.
- Encourage our loved ones to carry a note detailing their health conditions, medicine and allergies, in case they suffer acute worsening of their condition.

- If a loved one is worried about breathing problems, we can provide help by
- Talking to them about their feelings. Ask if they have something to say or ask them how they are feeling. Or provide physical comfort by holding a hand, a shoulder or giving them a head massage.
- Distract them with something that they like or bring something they like to keep them busy and occupied.
- If the loved one won't talk with us, give them space. Sometimes it is better to give them some time alone and approach later.
- Help them shift position to make breathing easier. Help them sit up straight as this position allows for deeper breaths.
- Use a fan to blow air over their face and body to help them relax and feel better.

Most importantly, don't lose the temper. Instead of scolding them or telling them what to do, remember they are probably scared and angry about what's happening to them. Be patient and sympathetic.

Managing breathing problems in the elderly

As the old saying goes, "prevention is better than cure". As loved ones age, caregivers can help by ensuring they follow important guidelines to reduce the risk of respiratory or cardiac issues.

- Stay away from drastic environmental changes such as temperature, moisture, pollution, pollen, smoke, chemical fragrance and dust.
- Make sure our loved ones eat regularly and healthily. Six smaller meals a day is better than three large ones. This not only helps in digestion but also supports immune system health. It is recommended to avoid spicy and oily food that may cause gas problems.

- Help them drink a lot of water and juices. If the patient is diabetic, keep a sugar count along with meals and juices. Encourage high-fiber food for healthy digestion.

- Daily exercise and physical activity not only maintain good health but can buoy the patient's spirits.

Pulmonary Rehab:

As per American Thoracic society: Pulmonary rehabilitation is a program of education and exercise that helps you manage your breathing problem, increase your stamina (energy) and decrease your breathlessness. The education part of the program teaches you to be "in charge" of your breathing instead of your breathing being in charge of you. You will learn how to pace your breathing with your activities, how to take your medicines and how to talk with your healthcare provider.

The program is conducted by a team of specialists. They who plan special exercises for patients to improve the strength of the muscles and breathing capacity.

Here are some points to consider while taking care of a loved one with a lung condition:

1. Is the shortness of breath and cough debilitating?
2. Does the patient need oxygen therapy?
3. Does the patient need BiPAP or trilogy machines?
4. Can the patient walk without assistance or without walkers?
5. Is there a need for wheelchair or motorized wheelchair?
6. Is the patient able to afford medicines?
7. Is the patient taking medication properly?

8. Is the patient bed bound?
9. Is the patient's life expectancy limited?
10. Does the patient need palliative or hospice care?
11. Does the patient have an associated heart condition, such as heart failure?
12. What is the role of lung rehabilitation?
13. Are the patient's flu and pneumonia vaccinations up to date? Influenza and pneumonia are very common among the elderly.

Oxygen therapy

Patients with advanced chronic lung disease often have low oxygen levels - there isn't enough oxygen in their blood for the body to operate properly. A person with low oxygen may have difficulty thinking and interpreting things clearly. Low oxygen level may cause dizziness and cause the heart to slow. If oxygen levels go too low, organs may start shutting down and eventually the body will die.

An oxygen machine can be used to treat or prevent these symptoms. The oxygen delivery system provides oxygen to the patient through a small tube that leads to the patient's nostrils. He or she doesn't need to do any extra effort to consume oxygen, just breathe normally.

There are three types of oxygen machines:

1. Concentrated gas -- Oxygen gas is compressed in metal canisters, which contain a flow regulator to determine the amount of oxygen flowing to the patient.

2. Liquid oxygen -- A storage tank is filled periodically with liquid oxygen. The tank is then warmed up which converts the liquid oxygen into gas form.

3. Oxygen concentrator -- this device pulls oxygen from the air and concentrates it inside its storage chamber.

Here are tips to consider when placing an oxygen machine in the home.

1. Oxygen is a flammable gas, so fire or any ignition materials should be kept out of the room containing the oxygen machine.

2. Naked wires should be taped or removed

3. The oxygen delivery system should be kept in a well-ventilated area to avoid a build-up of pure oxygen in the room, which would increase the probability of a fire.

The oxygen provided at home is calculated in LPM (liters per minute). An oxygen prescription generally ranges between 1 to 10 liters per minute depending upon the need of the patient. More than 6 liters per minute is a red flag; anything above this level is an indication that the patient would not be able to survive without oxygen therapy.

Cancer

Cancer is a condition in which our body keeps on producing defective cells. This action squeezes out healthy cells and also causes organ dysfunction. It is one of the worst degenerative diseases we can contract, because it causes great suffering and often is fatal.

Cancer is the second leading cause of death worldwide, according to the medical website _cancer.org_. Lung, prostate and colorectal cancer are the top causes of cancer death in men while lung, breast and colorectal cancer are leading causes of cancer death in women.

Many cancers are curable, even in the elderly. The surgery and other treatments can result in improved quality of life even if the objective of surgery is not to increase the expected life span.

Cancer is not just a physical disease. It carries the stigma which is mental and emotional effects as well. Patients need a lot of help while coping with cancer. As with many other chronic conditions, some of the elderly will not want to ask for help while they're coping with cancer. They don't want to be bothersome or a burden to their loved ones. Many elderly loved ones become frail but still want to do things by themselves. It's up to that support network to see the need for help and to provide it without waiting to be asked.

Risk factors

Unhealthy habits such as smoking, drinking, maintaining a poor diet, lack of exercise, obesity and poor sleeping habits all contribute to the risk of developing cancer. A healthy lifestyle not only develops muscle strength, controls diabetes, controls blood pressure and increases blood oxygen level, but can also help their emotional well-being.

Being healthy reduces a person's risk of cancer; if cancer develops, that same lifestyle increases the chance of surviving it. The presence of problems such as diabetes, vascular disease or impaired body functioning increases the risk of infection for the individual and can be an important obstacle during the person's recovery stage. Such conditions will not only slow the recovery process, they may result in incurable side effects.

Cancer treatment

Cancer can be curable despite the age of the patient or the stage of the cancer. The severity of the cancer can be reduced with the right treatment and therapy. Therefore, a caregiver needs to be very cautious and do periodic check-ups of their loved ones to make sure they are healthy and do not develop any kind of cancer related complications.

The presence of other chronic and uncontrolled problems like diabetes, vascular disease, and impaired body functioning increases the risk of complications for the individual and can be an important obstacle during the person's recovery stage.

One of the important things that should be done during long term cancer treatment is that the patient should have the love, care and support from close friends and family members as it is quite essential for the emotional health of the patient. Sometimes emotional support is more important and without it the patient might not be able to recover from his/her current situation.

How to help a loved one with cancer

Three out of every four families will have a member diagnosed with cancer. If our family is one, there are many ways for family and friends to help. No one is expecting us to cure our loved one's cancer, but "being there" can make a world of difference. Lend an ear or offer a shoulder for comfort. Those can be as important as driving our loved one to treatment.

1. Instead of rushing into a decision, caregivers should help their loved ones in getting the second opinion, if they are not satisfied.
2. Do some research. Learn about their illness and the treatment options.
3. Don't rule out complementary therapies such as massages, fitness programs, a short vacation or yoga. These can help our loved one to reconnect to society and his or her daily routine.
4. Help our loved ones get the best possible treatment, making sure they are in a quality medical facility which caters to their needs.
5. Remember the little things. Cook dinner or do a load of laundry.
6. Make them realize they are not forgotten. Drop by with a dozen cookies or a bouquet of flowers.

Be prepared for the possibility of mood swings. As treatments take a physical and emotional toll, our loved one may suffer rage or depression, which can cause confusion or poor decision-making.

When a loved one is diagnosed with cancer the family as a group should develop a plan of action. Talking through these questions can help:

1. Do we need a second opinion?
2. What is the prognosis?
3. What treatment is available?
4. What are the side effects of the treatment?
5. How long is the treatment?
6. If the cancer goes into remission, will it come back?

The next discussion should be about treatment options:

1. Is my role to provide emotional care only?
2. Am I physically able to care for my loved one?
3. Can he or she live at home?
4. Does the patient need financial support?
5. How often will the patient need to visit the doctor or get admitted to the hospital?
6. Does the patient get enough rest?
7. Does the patient need help with anxiety and/or depression?
8. Is there anything else I can do to improve his or her quality of life?
9. Does he or she need palliative care?
10. Does he or she need hospice care?
11. Does the patient need funeral arrangements?

Neurological Disorders

Aging affects nearly every organ in our body, brain and nervous system are no exception. Impairments that affect our brain or nervous system include; stroke, multiple sclerosis (MS) or Parkinson's disease etc.

Stroke

A stroke is a dangerous, potentially life-threatening event in which the blood supply to the brain is interrupted. It can be caused by blockage of a blood vessel or by a vessel rupture within the brain. According to the Centers for Disease Control and Prevention (CDC), about 795,000 Americans suffer a stroke and 140,000 die from a stroke annually, making it the fifth-leading cause of death in the U.S. Strokes are one of the most common causes of disability among the elderly and affects the mobility of more than half of all stroke survivors.

<u>Recognize a stroke</u>

If a loved one suffers a stroke, getting treatment quickly is critical. If the stroke is caused by a clot, damage will continue to grow until the clot is removed. If a blood vessel ruptures, again damage will continue to grow until it is repaired. The signs and symptoms of stroke are very characteristic and can be spotted by remembering to BE FAST:

B – Balance (Loss of balance.)

E – Eyes (Loss of vision or blurred vision.)

F – Face drooping (Face looks uneven, one side of the face droops or sags)

A – Arms (Arm or leg weakness or one side of the body weakens).

S – Speech (Difficulty in speaking or slurred speech).

T – Time is critical (Call 911 immediately)

Stroke can occur at any age, but the risk of stroke increases as you age. The most common risk factors are considered to be:

- High blood pressure
- High cholesterol levels
- Smoking
- Obesity
- Diabetes

Fortunately, all these risk factors can be controlled. Maintaining a healthy diet, keeping active and avoiding alcohol and smoking are great ways to lower chances for stroke.

Multiple sclerosis

Multiple sclerosis or MS is a potentially disabling disease that affects the brain and the spinal cord. The nerves of the human body are covered with a protective sheath known as the myelin sheath. In MS, the immune system of the body attacks the myelin sheath, disrupting communication between the brain and the rest of the body. Depending on the severity and location of the affected nerves, MS can exhibit different symptoms which will worsen over time:

- Movement – Weakness or numbness of limbs on one side of the body; electric-shock-like sensation when moving the neck; tremors and problems walking.
- Vision – Double vision; blurred vision; partial or total loss of vision in one eye; and pain during eye movements.

- Other functions – Speech problems; problems in thought process; in sexual functions; in bowel and bladder function; and tingling sensation in different parts of the body.

According to a study organized by the National Multiple Sclerosis Society (NMSS), 947,000 Americans suffer from MS. Although the cause is not known, it is believed that genetics and environmental factors play a role.

Common risk factors include:

Age -- the risk increases with age

Gender -- Women are more likely to suffer MS than men

Family history increases the risk

Certain infections such Epstein-Barr are linked to MS

Ethnicity -- Caucasians are more likely to suffer MS then other ethnicities

Smoking

Parkinson's disease

Parkinson's disease is another common neurological disorder that affects elderly people. It affects more than 1 percent of the elderly population and causes progressive neurological deterioration. Although the progression of Parkinson's disease can be slowed, it cannot be healed. There is no definite treatment recognized to date, but there are medications to help manage the symptoms.

About 50,000 Americans are diagnosed with Parkinson's disease every year. Currently about half a million people suffer from this condition. The risk of Parkinson's disease increases with age and the average age of onset is regarded as 60 years. It is very uncommon to find this condition among younger individuals, especially in those younger than 40.

This neurological condition mainly affects movement. The symptoms may start as barely noticeable tremors on one side of the body. It will progress over time to affect both sides. The side of the body that is affected first will usually remain worse even when both sides of the body are affected. Over time, the symptoms will worsen, with the patient ultimately confined to a wheelchair.

The most common symptoms of Parkinson's disease are:

Tremors – shaking movements that usually begin in one hand and are present even at rest.

Slowed movement – This condition will slow your movements making easy daily tasks difficult and time-consuming. Gait will be changed as well.

Rigid muscles – It might limit the movements

Impaired posture and body balance – A stooped posture is common

Decreased ability to perform unconscious movements such as smiling and blinking

Speech and writing changes

Difficulty swallowing

Memory Loss

The cause of Parkinson's disease is not yet known; as with MS, genetics and environmental factors appear to be responsible.

A healthy lifestyle appears to reduce the risk of contracting Parkinson's.

Preparing for and dealing with neurological disorder

The neurological problems can be as simple as a tiny stroke, from which the patient recovers completely or it can be a debilitating disease that leaves them bed-bound. Either way, there are some things to keep in mind:

- We need to make sure the whole family understands the effects and prognosis of the disease process
- We need to be very patient as neurological problems will cause a lot of anxiety for our loved ones
- We need to help them find the proper care which may include finding the right rehab facility or finding the right home health service for physical therapy
- We should get ready to spend more time with the loved ones.
- We have to ask them repeatedly about their needs and wants. Sometimes our loved ones may not be able to understand, so we may have to guess, or ask the nurses, doctors and other healthcare staff
- We should be willing to find a skilled nursing facility for them if needed
- In the most advanced stages, the emotional help which our elderly loved ones will need will increase exponentially. That is the time they will need our help the most. They may have behavioral issues and may need psychological and psychiatric help. We will need to understand that what they are going through has made them helpless.
- During the advanced stages doctors may suggest tube feedings. At that time one person may not be able to understand. The whole family needs to get together and discuss the prognosis and risks and

benefits of tube feeding with the doctor. Is it necessary? Is it going to increase the life expectancy? Is it going to improve the quality of life? Is it safe? Does it cause more benefits than harm?

- We have to see whether our loved ones have advanced care directives. We will need a family meeting for advanced care directives if our loved ones are not mentally capable of making those decisions. We will need to understand the difference between DNR and FULL CODE. We may have to discuss the implications of advance care directives, on lives of our elderly loved ones.

- There will be a time, when we will have to discuss palliative care and hospice. We have to get ready for it, emotionally and mentally.

Yes, these situations are tough. Some of us may think that we are not able to make those decisions due to their nature, but we will still have to make these decisions any way. Planning well ahead of time and slowly getting ourselves ready may help us to some extent. We may have to do one small thing at a time and move to the next one slowly. We may have to seek the help of the healthcare staff, friends, pastor etc. I can't say tough it up and make the decision. No, it is not easy.

Later on, we will discuss all the emotions caretakers go through and how to cope with those.

PART III

PHYSICAL CONDITION OF THE ELDERLY LOVED ONES

Physical Condition and Daily Living

The physical condition of older adults is an integral part of the decision-making process. The physical condition of the elderly loved one is more visible relative to a mental condition, however, that does not necessarily make the decision any easier to make.

Just as how a physically fit but mentally unstable elderly poses a danger to themselves and others, a patient may be mentally fit but may have physical problems. These physical challenges may impact their standard of living enough to prompt a tough decision needing to be made. These are the times that would require difficult decisions to be made that may involve calling for help.

Therefore, let us further dissect the factors we should take into consideration when assessing the physical condition of the elderly.

Here are several factors to consider when assessing the physical condition of the elderly:

Mobility

Good mobility refers to the loved one's ability to move about freely and easily without assistance.

<u>Walking</u>

The ability to walk freely allows us to examine the most basic indicator of physical health. If the elderly loved ones have difficulty walking 20 feet, then they will likely have difficulty performing everyday tasks, that impact on the quality of life at home.

The lack of ability to walk without assistance could pose a risk to their well-being as the chance of experiencing falls may rise. In these types of cases where a loved one faces difficulty in walking, we may have to intervene and consider asking them to use a type of wheelchair or walker for extended periods of movement. However, it is important that we do not impose these decisions on the elderly.

We must employ empathy and put ourselves in their shoes. It is imperative that we explain to them the reasons behind the potential solutions and how those solutions would benefit our loved ones. We must treat them how we would want to be treated in this type of difficult situation.

Elderly loved one with difficulty in walking may be asked to use walkers or canes so that they can have the appropriate support. With this additional support, many elderly loved ones are able to improve their mobility significantly, as well as protect themselves from any potential risk for falls.

However, many older people ignore these devices as they believe that they are fine. Here, the problem becomes both physical and mental and increases the dangers that they face every day. They may now experience falls, which at an elderly age can lead to many calamities such as fractures and could make their physical condition even worse. Elderly loved ones on blood thinning medications are more prone to injuries from falls and it is important to provide them with the correct support needed.

In these types of cases, we must talk to our loved ones and try to understand their perspective while also making sure that we get our point across and convince them of the importance of using canes or walkers.

Use of a wheelchair

An elderly loved one who is wheelchair bound will face difficulties living at home without the proper level of care. A wheelchair-bound patient usually requires 24/7 care as they are unable to properly take care of themselves.

The decision here involves multiple difficult decisions. Should we keep our loved one at home or place them in a long-term care facility? If we decide to keep them at home, should we hire personal care or assistance?

These decisions require us to account for how much time we can provide in taking care of our loved ones and the level of care they need. We need to make sure that they are provided with a safe environment.

Even a wheelchair-bound loved one will have various limits to their mobility. Some may be unable to move in and out of the chair themselves. Other individuals will not be able to move the chair by themselves at all. In these cases, our elderly loved one might need an automatic wheelchair. There are then many subsequent difficult decisions on whether a family can afford an automatic wheelchair - even with insurance - or if the loved one should be placed in a long-term care facility.

On the other hand, some may use it to improve the level of comfort in their lives and are able to get in and out or move about in the chair on their own.

One of my patients was a wheelchair-bound woman who was fine mentally but had physical problems that prevented her from moving about on her own. She had two very caring daughters who were able to be with her from 1 to 8 p.m. and 8 p.m. to 8 a.m. But she was alone for a five-hour stretch from 8 a.m. to 1 p.m., when both daughters had to be at work. The family couldn't afford to hire in-home help for her.

She became lonely and depressed and suffered physically because she was unable to change her own diapers and sometimes sat in her own waste for hours until her daughter arrived. She began suffering extremely painful urinary tract infections. The daughters weren't able to fully provide for her needs and had to consider a nursing home to ensure their mother received the constant care she needed.

In cases like this, the family has to decide that maybe a nursing home would be a good option due to the constant care that their mother would receive there. She may have a better quality of life in a long term facility.

<u>Mobility in bed-bound patients</u>

One of the most difficult situations a family will face is when a loved one becomes bedridden. It may be difficult to provide the level of care needed if the patient wants to remain in his or her home. The patient and his or her loved ones need to decide the best location for the patient to receive care.

As with a wheelchair-bound patient, the level of self-care that bed-bound patients can manage can vary widely. Some can sit up and perform a fair number of actions, such as feeding themselves and changing their clothes or diapers. Such patients might be cared for in their home.

On the other hand, some bedridden patients need assistance to turn over in bed. Even if the family can provide care, they must consider potential problems that could occur, such as pressure sores or decubitus ulcers. These are caused by long periods of lying down or sitting stationary in a single position. This usually occurs on tissue and skin that covers the bony areas of your body. The area experiences poor circulation. This, combined with wear and tear on the skin, causes ulcers that are extremely painful and infectious. These sores can lead to sepsis which can be fatal. Caretakers need to constantly move bedridden patients and take extra care in activities such as dressing.

Bedridden people also face the risk of pneumonia, constipation, contractures, deformity of muscles and joints, urinary tract infections and depression.

The physical condition that leads to a bedridden loved one can be detrimental for mental health as well. Being unable to move much at all often brings a feeling a sense of helplessness. This is a potential reason why we would consider not sending a loved one to a nursing home, as they may feel lonely there.

Human interaction, especially with family for many older adults, is an important factor that keeps these individuals mental health strong. These risks must be weighed within the decision-making process when dealing with a bedridden loved one.

We must also provide immediate relief for any pain so that our loved ones can breathe properly. Urinary tract infections can be prevented by using manual emptying, timely changing of unclean underwear/diapers, and providing an adequate amount of hydration.

Now keeping all these in mind, we must decide which is the best way to provide comfort to our loved one and if whether we would be able to do enough ourselves at home to minimize the risks of these potential complications occurring.

Occurrence of falls in loved ones

The most prevalent cause of physical injury in the elderly is falling and it can lead to a host of long-term complications. Around 10% of falls in the elderly cause major injuries such as fractures and intracranial injuries.

In the United States, among those aged 65-74, falls cause 48% of unintentional nonfatal injuries, and 23.4% of unintentional fatal injuries. These proportions are even higher among those 75 years and older, in whom falls make up 71.2% of unintentional nonfatal injuries and 39.3% of unintentional fatal injuries. More than a third of the population 65 years of age or older falls each year, and half of these falls are recurrent. As the U.S. population ages, the total direct cost for falls is expected to be $43.8 billion by the year 2020.

There are certain risk factors that contribute to an increased probability of falls. These include, but are not limited to, age greater than 85 years, stroke, Parkinson's disease, arthritis, fractures, dementia, diabetes, vitamin D deficiency, anemia, arrhythmias, neuropathy, impaired vision/hearing, recent hospital discharge, higher body mass index, poor sleep/obstructive sleep apnea, and urinary incontinence.

Some medications increase the risk of falls in patients. These include psychiatric meds, narcotic pain meds, blood pressure medicines, benzodiazepines etc. As mentioned earlier, blood thinning medications should also be avoided in elderly patients unless they are absolutely necessary as they also increase the probability of injuries from falls.

Therefore, we must evaluate the cost and benefits of using medications that may cause falls as a side effect. It is important to consult with a doctor as to whether a medication is necessary and consider that maybe our loved one's quality of life would be better without it.

There are several types of tests doctors can perform to identify balance impairments, gait abnormalities and detecting fall risk.

Our goal is to provide a safe environment for our loved ones to live in. A lot of elderly loved one's experience falls in the bathroom due to slipping or tripping. Wet floors and a lack of support in bathrooms can lead to falls. Occupational therapists can play a big role in making sure that homes are as "older adult friendly" as possible.

One of my patients told me about having experienced a fall in her bathtub and could not move for many hours because she was living alone. Her daughter was calling her since the morning and when she didn't pick up, the daughter asked the neighbors to check up on her. The neighbors were only able check several hours later and found her in the bathtub - fallen and unable to get up.

As a result, in situations like this where the mother is prone to falls, a family should avoid letting her live alone. Other ways to make the environment safer from falls is to add handlebars beside bathtubs and toilets, improve lighting, and use fall-alert bracelets and bed alarms. Apple watch also has a fall alert feature in it now.

We must assess the risks of injury from falls to make an informed decision. The frailty of a loved one will determine how much damage a potential fall may cause them.

The frailty of an elderly loved ones may be measured by their ability to do everyday tasks such as carrying a bag of groceries and walking up & downstairs. Keeping this in mind, we must decide what steps we need to take to provide the correct level of care and attention to our loved one and if we can provide the care they need.

Continence

Continence refers to the ability of a person to control the movement of their bowels and bladders. Incontinence can have a significant impact on the quality of lives of the elderly loved ones. It becomes our responsibility to help them make the best decisions to minimize any sort of discomfort caused to them by continence issues.

There are two types of incontinence that could occur: Incontinence of the bladder and incontinence of the bowels.

Urinary incontinence refers to one's inability to control the functioning of their bladder. There are various causes of urinary incontinence that may develop with age and many seniors suffer from it. Causes may include (but are not limited to):

- A weak or an overactive bladder that is unable to hold urine.
- Possible damage to nerve controls of the bladder due to Parkinson's, MS or other diseases
- Possible damage to spinal cord or nerves that control bladder function
- Enlarged prostate in men.

There are several types of urinary incontinence and it is important to discuss with the physician to find the best method to identify and counteract the specific type our loved one suffers from. The various types are:

- Functional incontinence: This occurs when loved ones face issues in mobility rather than problems with their bladder function. This means that they have difficulty actually getting to the bathroom and thus they are reluctant to be too far from a restroom at any one point in time
- Overflow incontinence: The bladder is never fully emptied upon trips to the restroom, thus it is always full, and the urine often leaks out. This is a problem more common in men.
- Urgency incontinence: The ability to 'contain' or 'hold-back' the urine is hampered thus they are unable to make it to the restroom

when a sudden urge arises to urinate. Individuals with cases like diabetes, MS or other issues often face this.

- Stress incontinence: Any sort of stress on the bladder from activities like coughing, sneezing, exercise or even laughing causes the bladder to leak. This usually occurs in women after menopause.

Fecal incontinence refers to the inability of a person to control their bowel movements. According to Foundation for Functional Gastrointestinal Disorders fecal incontinence affects around 17 million people in the USA

In addition, fecal incontinence is one of the most common reasons due to which the older people are admitted to nursing homes and it's estimated around a third of the elderly in nursing homes have it.

Those suffering from fecal incontinence often have impaired rectal sensation. It means that they do not have awareness of the presence of stool in the rectum and thus, by the time they realize the need to defecate, the stool leaks.

Fecal incontinence can have various causes and the identification of the cause is an important step to providing the correct care to our loved one. Following are the most common causes of fecal incontinence:

Hemorrhoid surgery

Dementia

Diarrhea

Constipation

A history of straining to pass stool

Any Damage to the muscles and nerves of anus, can cause incontinence

Stroke

Diabetes

Surgery

Multiple sclerosis

Spinal cord injury

Rectal change due to rectal and pelvic cancer

Reduced physical activity

Each cause requires a different method of treatment. Symptoms of some may be reduced through home care such as through proper exercise, diet, hygiene or giving appropriate time to toileting. Other serious causes would require methods like bowel training, medication, or even surgery.

Therefore, by identifying the cause of fecal incontinence and the appropriate treatment method, we can work towards making the best decision for our elderly loved ones. We must remember that it is important to talk with our loved ones and work with them in making any sort of decision.

Many older people have urinary or bowel incontinence and thus they require pull-ups/diapers. This, though a nuisance, does not significantly impact their quality of life if they are able to change the diapers themselves.

The risk of developing diseases or infection increases drastically as they may end up wearing the diapers or pull-ups longer than they should. The risk of urinary infections, especially in females, goes up significantly and can lead to severe suffering.

The mental anguish to loved ones who suffer from incontinence could also be significant. The shame that accompanies uncontrollable bladder or bowel movement can cause great distress amongst loved ones. It is our job to eliminate this shame and make them understand that they are not at fault in this situation and what they are going through is entirely normal.

Over half of the elderly population has some form of incontinence; however, it is still understandable that the loved ones would not want to be seen in their condition. This can lead to a state of social seclusion, which could be potentially very harmful in any age - but especially in older adults. In this situation our loved may need social, psychological and physical support. Many elderly don't want to go out of their homes due to fecal incontinence.

Everyday activities

Quality of life for our loved one can be affected by any sort of difficulties in doing everyday activities. We must take these into consideration when trying to provide the best care for them.

Feeding difficulties in elderly loved ones:

Various problems and disabilities may hamper the ability of a loved one to feed themselves. We need to evaluate a number of factors to make the best decision in regard to providing the quality care for them. We must evaluate the nature of the problem that holds them back from feeding themselves.

Mental issues such as dementia can leave a patient incapable of doing tasks such as eating properly and at the right times. Cases like these require that we step in and give elderly loved ones the suitable support that they need.

Dementia can cause various problems in feeding, including confusion or lack of coordination while eating. We may, for example, see a loved one trying to drink food or trying to use a knife like a spoon. We might also notice behavioral changes such as sudden dislike or distaste towards food that they previously may have liked.

There are many steps we can take to manage feeding difficulties in patients with dementia. We must provide a set routine and ensure that mealtimes are set for certain times in a day. We should not rush mealtimes and allow them to take as long as they need. Allowing our loved ones to relax while eating in a quiet and calm environment can also be quite beneficial

As their caregivers, we must remain calm even when an elderly loved one with dementia faces feeding difficulties, as that uneasy feeling can be transferred onto them and make the situation worse.

We must do our best to let them do the most they can. If we see them having difficulties give them gentle hints and prompts on what to do and if this does not work, then we may load their spoon or fork for them. While eating, tell them about what they're eating so that they may recognize the different types of food. Finger foods are often a great strategy to simplify the feeding process.

<u>Grooming difficulties in elderly loved ones:</u>

If the elderly loved one is beginning to show signs of poor personal hygiene, it is very often an indicator that it may be time to step in and provide them with some sort of assistance. This may mean either a higher intensity of care at home or a move into a nursing home or assisted living.

As our loved one's age, it is common for menial everyday tasks to become an exhaustive effort. It is our job, as their family and caretakers, to directly address this issue (though it is possibly difficult & painful to do so) before it's too late.

The first step is to have a direct conversation with our loved one. Receiving help from others can be embarrassing for loved ones and it's important to talk to them or involve a doctor in the conversation to counter their feelings of humiliation.

The inability to groom oneself isn't necessarily reason enough for us to get in contact with the nursing home. However, this difficulty may surface in combination with a number of other problems and so we need to assess the situation with a clear mind and make the decision that is best for them.

Once I had a elderly patient visit me in the office. She was talking fine, and she was also mentally healthy. She did not believe that there were any issues with her. She was living alone, and her daughter was in another city. However, I noticed she was looking scruffier than usual, so I inquired about her grooming practices. The last time she had taken a bath was one week prior to visit and she eventually admitted she no longer had the energy to maintain the same grooming routine as before. I immediately contacted her daughter, and now they live together. With her daughter's assistance in grooming, the older adult is able to enjoy her home.

This could potentially have been dangerous as poor hygiene could have resulted in various medical problems, which are very problematic in the elderly.

If we are acting as a caretaker for a elderly loved one who has difficulty in grooming themselves, then we may find it useful to consider these tips:

- We may have to help our loved ones in bathing and still respect their privacy
- If the elderly loved ones want to wear the same clothes repeatedly then buy 2-3 similar outfits.

- Elderly loved ones don't need to take a bath daily if they don't want to. Bathing daily can lead to dry skin
- Clean the skin folds in a good way, as a lot of germs grow in skin folds, groin area and arm pits. Clean with soap and water then dry it properly by patting with towel.
- Dental and oral hygiene needs to be taken care of as well. Use electronic toothbrushes, encourage the use of mouthwash and help them select the optimal toothpaste and toothbrush.

Difficulties in use of bathrooms/restrooms:

Falls may be common in elderly loved ones who go to the restroom in a rush or when they sit or stand from the toilet due to volatility in blood pressure. This may happen even in loved ones who are mentally and physically independent.

Again, as mentioned before, the most important thing here is clear communication between us and our loved one. Use short concise suggestions to encourage our loved one to do as much as they can by themselves. Give them directions like "The toilet seat is right behind you. Sit down slowly in a squat".

Encourage them to set routines of visiting the bathroom, after meals, for example, to reduce the chances of accidents.

As with when assisting loved ones in grooming, receiving help from others when going to the toilet can cause great shame in our loved ones. We need to keep a clear dialogue with them and the doctor to minimize such feelings and make them as comfortable as possible.

Though most issues related to going to the bathroom can be resolved at home through better care and installation of disabled supporting infrastructure, we may need to consider nursing homes or assisted living in some severe cases.

Furthermore, we must ask the following question: 'Does patient need help with changing diapers?'.

Usually, loved ones suffering from bladder or bowel incontinence have to wear adult diapers as a tool for providing them a sense of comfort and relief. It alleviates the stress of potentially having an accident spoiling their clothes. They're also convenient and thin - thus not noticeable through clothing.

The act of wearing diapers rarely serves as an inconvenience to our loved ones and helps them significantly. However, problems arise when the elderly have difficulties in changing their adult diapers. The level of care they now require, increases. We must look at the reason. Why are they unable to change their diapers. Are they bedbound due to a physical disability? Are they suffering from dementia? Or any other reason. Try to solve the problem, if we can.

We must also consider the level of care and time we can give, as a family, to our loved ones. An older adult unable to change their diapers on their own will likely require someone to be within calling distance for the majority of the day, and they cannot be left alone for long.

If we are unable to be with them during the day, then it may be time to have a sitter with them, if sitter is not possible then assisted living or skilled nursing home can be a good choice.

A patient of mine was an elderly mother with dementia. Her family came to me and told me that she had been treating their whole home as a sort of 'open toilet'. She would urinate and move her bowels anywhere she wanted throughout the house and it had become almost impossible for the family to manage the situation. Both the mother and the family members had a poor quality of life at home. *I suggested that he best choice for both parties, mother as well as the family, was to move mom into skilled nursing facility, where she could get the proper care she needed. This was indeed very difficult and painful for the family, but later on they were happy that they made a good choice.*

Following tips may help when changing diapers if the patient is at home:

- Make sure to do the process in the most private area possible to avoid our loved one feeling any embarrassment.

- Use disposable gloves and place the dirty clothing in a separate laundry bag.

- Don't be hesitant to use multiple wet wipes to clean the area, as we need to make sure the area is completely clean to avoid infections.

- Roll the loved one to their side when taking the diaper off and fold the diaper to get as much of the stool and urine as possible.

- Make sure to always check for signs of irritation or rash after we finish cleaning and apply diaper cream.

- Clean the area once we are done and trash anything that has been used.

Many a times if we are going out to eat or shop, we may have to carry a hand bag for our elderly loved ones. In this bag we can put diapers and an extra set of clothes, just like the way parents carry a bag for their infants and toddlers.

Access to 3 meals a day

The State of Senior Hunger in America annual report series, released in 2019 using 2017 data, found that 5.5 million seniors, or 7.7% of the senior population, were food insecure in 2017. According to feedingamerica.org, the rate of food insecurity among seniors is lower in recent years but remains significantly higher than it was in 2007.

In the United States of America alone, every 1 in 7 elderly is in threat of hunger according to the National Foundation to end senior hunger.

Good nutrition is an important part of the life of any person and with age that importance only increases. Bad nutrition can become the root cause of many bigger complications and can effectively destroy the life of a loved one, over time. Many a times providing the good quality, correct level, and timely nutrition to a loved one becomes our responsibility as they do not have the capacity to do it themselves.

It is not only important to provide meals at the right times of the day and at the right quantity, but also important that we provide nutrition that is correct for them. For example, If our loved one has diabetes, their diet will have to be optimized to keep their blood sugar levels in control. If they have heart failure then their salt intake needs to be controlled etc.

There are a few challenges an elderly can face due to old age that disrupt proper nutrition

As we age we have decreased sensitivity, which includes the sense of taste. This means that our loved one could potentially face difficulty in differentiating between fresh food and spoiled food. This could be potentially very dangerous to health as an elderly immune system is already weak and spoiled food could have a detrimental effect. Therefore, it is important that we take responsibility to provide fresh food to them regularly or arrange for them to only eat fresh healthy food.

- ✓ A lack of finances is a major concern among the elderly which may cause them to compromise on their nutrition. We must communicate to them the importance of good nutrition and provide them some financial assistance or find an appropriate alternative.

- ✓ Side effects of medications the elderly loved ones take, can also affect their nutrition. This is due to the fact that some medicines can cause nausea, a change in perception of food tastes or reduced appetite.

- ✓ Many elderly loved ones may also have bad dental health, as age can cause issues such as receding gums or missing teeth, which can lead to jaw pain or sores in their mouth. This can cause the act of eating to become painful and uncomfortable. The elderly loved ones may become discouraged to eat the right amount of food due to this problem. We must consult a dentist to alleviate our loved one's pain as much as possible and cook food that is relatively easy to chew so that they do not have to exert as much effort.

Another potential hindrance faced by elderly loved ones is a lack of proper transport that would allow them to go to a grocery store and shop for fresh groceries. Extreme weather conditions can make this activity even more difficult. Here, we can be the one to provide them with fresh groceries by getting them ourselves or find an alternative such as asking a neighbor to do so if our parents live alone. We may hire help. Nowadays, there are services like Ubereats and Doordash which help in getting groceries or cooked meals from restaurants delivered. There are also many grocery stores who deliver groceries and a whole variety of other stuff.

- ✓ Physical disabilities or problems such as arthritis and the overall physical weakness that comes with age can make the simple function of preparing food and feeding oneself appear extremely difficult. We should encourage our loved ones to work as much as they can themselves, however, it is important they don't overexert themselves, so we need to provide them with assistance in cooking or find someone to do so.

- ✓ Alzheimer's disease and loss of memory due to any kind of dementia may pose a challenge in regard to nutrition. It is easy for someone suffering from dementia to forget to buy fresh groceries or even forget to eat a meal altogether. This poses a danger to their health and thus they require a greater level of care.

  Dementia patients will require more assistance in feeding; thus we may want to consider home health, sitters at home, assisted living or nursing homes depending on the intensity of memory loss and help they need.

- ✓ Finally, age can bring about a host of mental changes and more often than not these changes have a negative impact. With time the older adults lose loving family members and friends, it becomes common that an elderly starts to feel lonely. A combination of factors can lead to depression and that can have a massive impact on the diet of our loved ones as they may not pay attention to their nutrition.

We should never be hesitant to acquire the help of a trusted therapist as mental health is extremely important in everyone, especially the elderly. If our loved one is starting to feel lonely then we may have to consider moving them to a nursing home where they can interact with other similar age people and get involved in group activities. However, that is not always enough and we as a family have to give them our time and interact with them regularly.

One of my patients was an elderly mom who was living alone in her home as her son and daughter were in another town. Her children came to me and told that their mom had not eaten properly for 2 days when they went to meet her and that she had been crying constantly in the house.

They were rightly very worried and lucky that no serious complication occurred in this dangerous situation. I suggested to them to see a psychologist friend of mine. Soon their mom was moved into assisted living where her mental health significantly improved as she made new friends. I also reminded her children that they needed to visit their mother more regularly.

Nowadays, it is understandable that some of us may be unable to provide our loved ones with the constant care they need. Many factors such as long working hours or working away from home may actually lead our elderly loved ones to become lonely and helpless. Therefore, we need to evaluate and see whether we are able to provide 3 healthy meals a day for our loved ones.

When we are unable to take out time to provide 3 meals a day for our loved ones or if our loved ones live on their own but are unable to properly provide for themselves, then Meal Delivery Service options can be a useful tool. This will allow us to provide quality food to our loved ones.

This is a good option to keep loved ones that do not require a high level of care away from nursing homes as they can have these meals at their home. Of course, the decision to keep a loved one at home is not entirely dependent on the availability of healthy food, but all other factors considered, this may be a great help.

In the United States, there are various options when looking for quality meal delivery services.

Meals on Wheels

According to the Meals on Wheels America website, it is the leadership organization supporting the more than 5,000 community-based programs across the country that are dedicated to addressing senior isolation and hunger. This network serves virtually every community in America and, along with more than two million staff and volunteers, delivers the nutritious meals, friendly visits and safety checks that enable America's seniors to live nourished lives with independence and dignity.

Churches and community services:

There are quite a few religious organizations and community centers, across the United States, who provide meal services to the senior citizens.

Ubereats, Grubhub, Doordash etc.

These services can help deliver food from our favorite restaurants.

These meal delivery services are great for elderly loved ones who live at home with family. It is great for the elderly who have a healthy social life. However, we need to realize that if our loved one was already living alone and was feeling lonely, then activating a meal delivery service which will further keep them at home may cause more harm than benefits. They may be better off in a long term assisted living facility or nursing home where they will have social interactions and proper meals, thus providing them with a better quality of life.

Medications

As we grow older the significance of medication in our lives begins to grow and it goes from being an occasional source of relief/cure to a regular part of everyday life. It is extremely important that our loved ones take the proper medications at the optimum time.

According to a study by the National Institutes of Health around 90% of the elderly take at least one prescription medication and over 40% of the elderly take five or more prescriptions.

Medications present a huge headache for caregivers. Not taking enough medications can cause the health of our loved one to deteriorate but taking too many unnecessary medications can also have detrimental effects.

Ability to afford medication

As per Bloomberg news report, Americans spend more on prescription drugs — average costs are about $1,200 per person per year — than anyone else in the world. This is in addition to the amount we spend on insurance premiums and other healthcare activities like going to the doctor. In this era of uncontrollable drug prices, it is becoming increasingly difficult for our loved ones to afford medicine.

The rising drug prices in the United States have become a huge headache for the whole population and its effects are being felt by the older people due to their limited income. A survey by AARP of nearly 2,000 adults age 50+ finds the vast majority — 81 percent — think drug prices are too high, and nearly 9 in 10 want politicians to do something about it.

Many elderly patients tell me that due to the rising drug prices they are unable to afford other medical care. Due to the high costs of prescription drugs, they are trying to avoid seeing a doctor unless they feel it absolutely necessary.

This is very dangerous as the elderly need to have good communication with a doctor. Even the smallest of the mishaps, can lead to something significant. It is our job as caregivers to make sure that our loved ones are visiting their doctors and keeping good communication with them as needed. This will help to maintain their quality of life.

There are some ways we can help our loved ones lighten the burden that prescription drugs put on their pockets.

- The first step is to have a conversation with the doctor to ask him to look at all the current drugs our elderly loved one is taking. The goal here is to identify any possible drugs that are unnecessary.

- Drugs that do not improve our elderly loved one's quality of life or improve life expectancy need to be cut out. Sometimes doctors may give medications even though there is little hope that they work and those medicines then end up costing a lot to patients.

The price of medicines vary a lot. Generic medicines sometimes are cheaper when we use services like www.Goodrx.com.

Medicare.gov suggests following tips to lower the prices of medicines in elderly loved one

- Consider switching to generics as most of them are cheaper than the name brand. Talk to the doctor about generic options are available to the patient.

- There are different types of drug plans and we need to help our elderly loved ones in choosing the right plan for them

- It will always be a good idea to call the medicare drug plan and ask them about suggestions to reduce the cost of medicine. Sometimes they provide a list of alternate medicines, which are cost efficient.

- Free Medication Therapy Management (MTM) program, is provided by insurance if the patient is in a medicare drug plan. This plan provides

A comprehensive review of your medications and the reasons why you take them.

An action plan to help you make the best use of your medications.

A written summary of your medication review with your doctor or pharmacist.

In conclusion, cut down on any unnecessary medications and make an effort to look for the cheapest retailer of the drugs. This may lead to cost saving and those funds can be utilized for other necessary activities.

Timely refilling of medications

If our loved ones do not refill their medications on time it can have detrimental effects as they could be left without important medications for vital periods of time. Any break or disruption in the treatment may cause setbacks to the patient. Some medicines are absolutely necessary for survival and not taking them can be catastrophic.

One of my patients with dementia was prescribed fluid pills for his heart failure, along with medicines for high blood pressure and diabetes. However, he was taking the medications on his own without the assistance of a family member. He took the medication and refilled normally for 2 months and so the family thought he was doing well on his own. However, after the second month, he completely forgot about the medication and did not remember to refill them. Within a month he was admitted to hospital with severe heart failure. Thankfully, he survived but there are so many who don't.

Some seniors may not be able to keep up with their medications as they may be using over 5 prescription medications at a time. They frequently forget when one particular medication needs to be refilled. Here, we should try and make sure that all the medications that our loved one is taking, are scheduled to be refilled at the same time to avoid complication and confusion.

If we observe that our elderly loved ones will not be able to take medicines properly by themselves, then we the caregivers may need to assume responsibility and help them refill and take medicines.

Unprecedented discontinuation of medicines

Many elderlies find adherence to medication very difficult. In fact, around half of the elderly population that take at least one medication find adherence difficult. There could be a host of reasons behind why a loved one would stop using medication and we may need to find the reasons and help them take the necessary medicines.

Elderly loved ones may themselves evaluate the risk and benefit of certain medicine and conclude that it does not benefit them enough, to continue using it. This kind of self-diagnosis and treatment is dangerous because even though the effects of a medication may not be seen immediately, it may play an important role in the long-term health of our loved one. For example, medication for control of diabetes, high blood pressure and high cholesterol may not have immediate effects but are necessary for great quality of life. These medicines improve the life expectancy.

In cases like these, we may provide constant care ourselves or provide periodic reminders about their medications throughout the day. However, if we are unable to do that, then it may be time to move our loved one to either assisted living or a nursing home where they can be attended to properly and receive the timely & correct dosage of medication.

I have a sign in my office which states "don't stop medications on your own, ask me". A big decision such as discontinuing medication is not one to be taken lightly based on one's own intuition. We need to encourage our loved ones to have conversations with their doctor to understand the benefit of each and every prescription of theirs. Patients may ask the doctor to review the medication periodically for any unnecessary prescription. If we feel that certain medicines are causing side effects, then we should talk to the doctor immediately.

The best remedy for most of these problems is to educate our elderly loved ones. We must work with the doctors to have conversations with the older adults about their medicines.

We may have to make the painful decision of moving them to assisted living or a nursing home if they suffer from problems such as dementia or are physically unable to take the medications themselves.

Missed/Skipped dosage of medications

Around 125,000 people in the USA pass away each annum due to improper dosage of drugs. In addition to that, around $100 billion extra is spent on hospitalizations and doctor visits which could have been preventable.

Worrisome side effects of medicines.

Some medications can have dangerous side effects and medication prescribed for one issue may actually end up causing or worsening another.

For example, if mom has knee pain then a doctor may prescribe Norco. However, Norco can cause one to feel dizzy and drowsy which may lead to falls. We all know how dangerous falls can be among the seniors.

- The danger of side effects increases as we get older. Many older adults will have one or more chronic illnesses and this means that they will receive different medications for each disease. The combination of certain medicines can cause confusion, dizziness, drowsiness and falls in the elderly loved ones.

It is important that we speak to doctors to make sure that our loved ones avoid medications that would adversely interact with one another and may cause major side effects. Clinicians are generally aware that medications can result in more severe adverse events among older adults, and the Beers Criteria have helped define those drugs that are best avoided in this population. Beers's list is a publication of potentially harmful medicines in elderly. This list is updated on a yearly basis and can help us make smart decisions for our loved ones.

- The risk of side effects can increase with food and drugs interactions. We usually know that we cannot take a particular medication with another medication, and the same can be said about food. Food and drug interactions are very important as the food we eat can have a massive effect on how a drug works.

For example, grapefruit juice can potentially lead to adverse reactions with over 85 different medications. Coumadin/Warfarin can be rendered useless when consumed alongside food rich in vitamin K. The solution here is to always be informed about the potential interactions of a particular medicine and to make sure our loved ones are also informed.

If the side effects of a particular medication are making the quality of life of our loved one significantly worse without providing a sufficient amount of benefit, then we need to discuss this with their doctor to either find an alternative medicine or to make the tough decision to stop the medicine altogether if it does not improve quality of life or life expectancy.

The biggest challenge I face in the nursing homes is reduction in the quantity or the doses of medicines. I round on the patients then order to stop few medicines, only to know next visit that medicines were never stopped as the family wanted to continue them.

So, many of the family members are reluctant. They don't want meds changed at all. Their argument "mom has been taking these for 20 years and they always work".

Instead of countering the doctor with the argument that "mom is on these meds for years" we should ask

Do these medicines hamper the safety and quality of life?

Do these medicines reduce the life expectancy of the loved ones?

Do these medicines decrease the appetite of the patient?

Do these medicines cause sleep problems in the patient?

Are these medicines detrimental to the health of the patient?

Do these medicines cause more falls?

Are these medicines habit forming?

Do these medicines cause constipation?

This way we will get a better and detailed response from doctors. The doses of medication are different for a toddler and an adult. Similarly doses of medication can be different for a 65 year old and 85 year old. Some elderly don't need too many medicines.

Summary

So in this section we discussed the physical limitations which the elderly may face. To summarize this, here is what we observe in our elderly loved ones. This should prompt us to take decision which may not look pleasant but will have long term benefits for our elderly loved ones.

- Mom is not able to walk properly, she may have a fall
- Mom is now wheelchair bound, but can propel the wheelchair
- Mom can't get out of the wheelchair on her own
- Mom is bed bound but she can help change and feed herself
- Due to her bed bound status mom has developing bed sores
- Mom was admitted to the hospital 3 times in last the 4 months with pneumonia, due to bed bound status and aspiration because of swallowing problems
- Mom can not turn in bed and can't even help in changing
- Mom is developing contractures in her arms and legs (severe stiffness of joints)
- Dad is unable to help mom
- I feel mom may fall while changing
- Mom had a fall in bathroom and she broke her hip
- Mom wears diapers now
- Mom can't change her diapers

- Mom is not interested in bathing
- Mom needs help in feeding
- Mom is losing weight as she doesn't cook often
- Mom doesn't have enough resources to buy her medicines
- Mom is skipping her medicines
- Mom doesn't refill her medicines properly
- Mom's insulin cost is 300 dollars a month

We can offer help to our elderly loved ones in the following ways. They may not like our help due to various factors, but sometimes we have to be firm for their safety, dignity and for them to have better quality of life.

As a care provider, we may have to offer/supply the following solutions to help our loved ones

- Visit their doctor with them and ask whether physical therapy will improve the functional status of our elderly loved one
- Help them install handrails in bathrooms
- Make sure that bathrooms are not slippery
- Help them use, cane or walker
- Try to help them with grooming and feeding, without making them feel bad about themselves
- Try to help them with meals, by cooking for them or by arranging with other resources
- Ask their doctors about their medicines
- Ask the doctors are there any medicines which mom can stop

- Ask the doctor if there are cheaper alternatives to the costly medicines

Many elderly loved ones don't ask for any kind of help. It becomes our responsibility to find the problems they are having and try to resolve the problem without getting too intrusive. We have to be careful as they don't want to lose their independence.

PART IV

Overall financial and social conditions of the caregivers

Factors Caretakers Must Consider About Themselves

Elderly care has transformed significantly in the United States. In the past, many families lived primarily in the same town or city, which provided a large support system for our elderly loved ones. As our loved ones age, taking appropriate care of them - with an emphasis on safety and comfort - requires increasingly more time.

Many times, as caretakers, we do not fully understand the challenges our elderly loved ones are going through. This lack of understanding then leads to assumptions on their situation, their desires, and what is best for them. When making difficult decisions about our loved ones, we must consider these various factors affecting us to ensure that we are making the best decision for the most important older adults in our life.

Time

Linda, 78, has been living with her son James, 44, for the past 10 years since her husband died. James and his wife, Sarah, have been Linda's only support system. James and Sarah both work full time and have noticed that Linda needs more help than in the past with day-to-day tasks. Even after work James and Sarah must take their children to soccer and basketball practice. Linda is beginning to feel lonelier. James isn't sure of what to do because he doesn't feel like he is giving his mother the time she deserves.

It is easy to see how busy our day-to-day lives have become. Most Americans who face these difficult decisions for their elderly loved ones are typically working at least 40 hours a week, most of the year. These individuals outside of work usually spend countless hours with their families. With these busy lives, it can be difficult to take full responsibility for our elderly loved ones and provide them the care that they need and deserve. Depending on care needed, it might be necessary for the various caretakers to be available 24/7. Consider these questions:

Do I have the time to help them with all of their meals?

Do I have the time to clean out their excreta if they are unable to do so?

Can someone be available within minutes when our loved one needs assistance?

Can I do all of these things my loved one needs along with the needs of my job and family?

Can I do enough to keep them engaged and not socially isolated?

Physical and Mental Condition of Caretaker

Susan, 64, primarily takes care of her 86-year old mother-in-law, Samantha. Susan is the sole caretaker as her husband usually travels out of town for work. A month ago, Susan fell in the bathroom and Samantha didn't have the strength to pick her up. With time, Susan has become increasingly preoccupied by the idea of Samantha falling.

<u>Physical capability of caretaker</u>

When considering the various pros and cons of a difficult decision we must make for our elderly loved one, we must look at our personal physical condition. This can be in the sense of physical strength as well as assisting them with mobility. Consider these questions:

Am I capable of helping them if they fall?

Will I be able to help them with routine tasks like grooming, moving, using the restroom, etc?

Will I be able to serve them the meals they want and need?

Can I clean out their waste if they need me to?

Mental issues of caretaker

Considering ourself as the 24/7 caregiver is difficult even if we are able to give elderly loved ones the time that they need. This can have a tremendous effect on mental health, which may be compounded by personal emotions of seeing our loved ones wither in front of our eyes. Consider these questions:

Is caring for my elderly loved one affecting my mental health and seriously detracting from my way of life?

Am I constantly stressed about my loved one?

Am I obsessed with the idea that I am still not enough to take care of them properly?

Is this sustainable for me? If not, how long can I do this before I must make another difficult decision.

Finances

The other day a patient's relative told me that she has not seen her mother in two years. It's because she lives in South Carolina and her mother is living at home in Owensboro, KY. She does not have resources or time to visit her mother, let alone take care of her. She is taking care of her daughter with cerebral palsy as well and works two jobs to support her family. So, she advised her mother to move to assisted living as she can afford it.

Are we able to provide financial support for our elderly loved ones? There are many costs associated with keeping our loved one at home as well as placing them in a long-term care facility where they will be comfortable. It is vital to fully explore what it would look like from a financial perspective before making any decisions.

Keeping an elderly loved one at Home

- Items to assist in mobility around the house
- Provision of three meals a day
- Provision of medicines and other supplies

Moving to Long Term Care Facility

- Will their health insurance cover all of the expenses for a facility where they will be happy?

Ultimately, financial resources are the backbone of most households and it is nearly impossible to make a decision without looking at the financial consequences.

Religious and Cultural Beliefs

Jeremy, 43, grew up with his grandparents living in the same house as him and his parents. His parents took care of his grandparents until he passed away. Now, his parents are approaching an age where they cannot live independently. Jeremy feels obligated to take his parents into his home due to his cultural upbringing even though he does not think he can give them the time they deserve.

A large contributing factor on difficult decisions may be based on religion or culture. It is normal and common for caretakers to believe that God has ordered and expects them to take care of their aging relatives. This means that taking care of our elderly loved ones is no longer just a moral responsibility; it is also a religious duty.

Biases

Before making any difficult decisions regarding care for our elderly loved ones, it is crucial for us to analyze our own biases and how they may be affecting our judgement. These biases may manifest through peer pressure, our feelings, any past promises, etc. Let's delve a little deeper into how we can analyze these biases to make the best choice for our loved ones.

<u>Peer Pressure</u>

We live in a society where peer and societal pressures have a great influence on our lives. We set our norms and morals according to society; therefore, most of our traditions are also dependant on the society we live in. All events are typically documented on social media, and if an event is not posted about then many people believe someone is trying to hide something. We are connected digitally and are judged at each and every step.

Caretakers often hesitate to put their loved ones in nursing homes or other long-term care facilities just because of the fear of society and what others will think.

It can be mistakenly perceived that opting to place our loved one in a long-term care facility is due to weakness and lack of integrity. Individuals often believe that making this decision is just forgoing the responsibility of taking care of someone who raised you.

It is crucial that we do some introspection on if any of these societal factors are influencing our decision. We must make decisions that first focus on the safety of our loved ones and second on their comfort and quality of life.

At the end of the day, we must all realize that It is better to have our loved ones somewhere other than home where they are getting three meals instead of having them at home where they are not getting proper meals and no one is there to clean them up.

Feelings of the Caretaker

One of my patients came to me and said that she had put her mother in the nursing home but now she is devastated with sadness and guilt. She was having some doubts and wanted to reverse her decision by bringing her mother back home

Are our personal feelings interfering with making a rational decision for our loved one? Some of the most common feelings individuals who must make difficult decisions must feel are those of guilt, sadness, loneliness, and many others.

Guilt

Robin 58, has promised her mother that she will never put mother in the nursing home. She promised it when she was herself 40-years-old and her mother was 70. Now, Mom is 88 and frail and Robin has severe arthritis which has limited her mobility. She is stressed that she can't break her promise and put her mother in a nursing home.

In the example like this we have to understand that we promised to keep them at home to provide good care and provide safety to our loved ones. So, our promise is more about care then keeping them at home. So, if we can't provide safety and care at home then there is no need to keep the promise which is harmful to our loved ones.

Most caretakers and their families who face the difficult decision of placing their loved one in a long-term care facility will deal with some degree of guilt. In fact, many people that decide to keep their family member at home make this decision to avoid the guilt.

Guilt is associated with performing a wrong deed or making a conscious mistake. If people do something bad, then they should be feel guilty or ashamed. But we are talking about taking care of elderly loved ones for their safety. We must make decisions that are best for our elderly loved ones.

One of the best ways to combat this guilt is making an informed, rational decision. This will provide constant reassurance to us as caretakers. If we are able to make these types of decisions, we will feel proud of our ourselves for not letting our personal emotions get in the way of our rational thinking and doing what is best for some of the most important individuals in our lives.

<u>Sadness</u>

Brenda Johnson wrote a book titled, "Once an Adult, Twice a Child" in regard to caring for the elderly and Alzheimer patients. This statement fully embodies the idea the deterioration that older adults face as they age. As a caretaker, it can be unfathomably difficult to watch someone who raised us slowly become unable to perform routine tasks. Simply observing this can cause a great deal of pain and sadness. When making difficult decisions, the sadness is often amplified because it may seem like we will not have any control in caring for our loved ones if we place them in a long-term care facility.

Despite the difficulty of dealing with our personal sadness in these decisions, it is crucial that we still make a rational decision. There are many ways to address this sadness if we do end up deciding that a long-term care facility is best. Mentality changes by viewing the decision as a positive act as well as consistent visits to help prevent social isolation have the potential to significantly reduce the sadness while also making sure that our loved ones are receiving the care that they deserve.

Loneliness

Even in old age, elderly loved ones provide a sense of comfort and belonging to their caretakers. If a caretaker is struggling with the decision of placing their loved one in a long-term care facility, then often times the caretaker also realizes that the loved one will no longer be a constant presence in their lives. It can be difficult dealing with the associated loneliness of not having someone like that easily accessible.

If we ever feel emotionally dependent on our loved ones, then it becomes even more important to acknowledge our dependency and how that may be affecting our decision. Even with this potential loneliness, it is crucial for us to emphasize the role of making the best decision for our loved one. This loneliness can always be combated by frequent visits to the loved one; however, an irrational decision may be much more detrimental in the long run for the entire family.

Social Support

"Are we making this decision based on only our own intuitions?"

"Do we trust explaining the situation to someone and having them assist us in figuring out the best way for us to support our family member?"

Some people don't want their elderly loved ones to be away from them because they are their only support system. They don't have many friends aside from their elderly loved ones. This is true for many men who can't separate from spouses due to fear of loneliness and this is true for some of the kids as well

Having social support from friends and family members out of the house can be a huge factor in deciding the best plan of action during a difficult decision. If we feel like we have a big support network that may be able to help with the decision or the subsequent steps after the decision, this can alleviate a lot of the pressure of the decision.

Selfishness

Many of the various factors we have discussed can be summarized by one word: selfishness. This selfishness may arise from any of the factors we have discussed like loneliness to the idea that caretakers believe others at long-term care facilities cannot take care of their loved one like they can. This selfishness is normal and common, but it does not mean we must not look past our personal desires in this situation. The big question becomes:

"Are we doing it 'to them' or 'for them.'"

We want to provide the best care possible, as they did for us when we were children.

What to Look For

In this book, we have discussed many issues that our elderly loved ones may face.

We have to empathize with elderly loved ones and help them make the decisions so that they are safe and live a dignified life. Quality of life has to be the utmost factor in deciding the care of elderly loved ones.

I am going to summarize the questions that we need to ask to help our elderly loved ones:

1. Look at the overall condition of the elderly loved one?
2. Are they safe in the current environment they live in?
3. Do they have three fresh meals a day?
4. Are they able to take care of their activities of daily living?
5. Are they able to walk around the house and outside the house?
6. Are they having falls?
7. Do they feel lonely?
8. Do they have a disease which is affecting them tremendously?
9. Are they extremely short of breath?
10. Are they sad and depressed?
11. Are they very anxious?
12. Do they have severe pain?
13. Do they have an incurable, severe disease?
14. Do they have a terminal disease?

15. Are we able to take care of them despite all our circumstances?

16. Are we satisfied with the care they're getting?

Asking the right questions will help us make the right decisions for our elderly loved ones. Many times, the solution which we will come up with will be hard on us and our loved ones. However, as long as we have made the decision to maintain their dignity, safety and quality of life in perspective, then we have done our best.

When we see any of the memory or behavior issues above in our elderly loved one then this is the time to talk to the primary care doctor or geriatrician. Take time to review the questions and information above to prepare and plan so that change will be easier for us and our loved one.

Further Reading:

On our website you can read more articles:
www.elderlylovedones.com

Connect with MD Mahesh Moolani:

If you have found the information in this book helpful, I would appreciate your feedback. You can leave a review on the following platforms:

Amazon

Goodreads

References

"10 Things You Should Know about LBD: Lewy Body Dementia Association." *10 Things You Should Know about LBD | Lewy Body Dementia Association*, www.lbda.org/go/10-things-you-should-know-about-lbd.

"Accidental Bowel Leakage: NAFC - URINARY INCONTINENCE EDUCATION: BLADDER HEALTH: NATIONAL ASSOCIATION FOR CONTINENCE." *URINARY INCONTINENCE EDUCATION | BLADDER HEALTH | NATIONAL ASSOCIATION FOR CONTINENCE*, www.nafc.org/bowel-health.

"Adherence Issues in Elderly Patients." *Pharmacy Times*, www.pharmacytimes.com/publications/issue/2011/january2011/rxfocus-0111.

Advanced Solutions International, Inc. *Suicide in the Elderly*, www.aamft.org/AAMFT/Consumer_Updates/Suicide_in_the_Elderly.aspx

Aisen1, Paul S., et al. "On the Path to 2025: Understanding the Alzheimer's Disease Continuum." *Alzheimer's Research & Therapy*, BioMed Central, 9 Aug. 2017, alzres.biomedcentral.com/articles/10.1186/s13195-017-0283-5.

American Psychological Association, American Psychological Association, www.apa.org/.

"Annual Meeting." *American Association for Geriatric Psychiatry*, www.aagponline.org/.

Bihari, Michael. "How Your Age Can Affect the Side Effects of Your Drugs." *Verywell Health*, Verywell Health, 10 Sept. 2019, www.verywellhealth.com/age-increases-risk-for-medication-side-effects-1123957.

"Birks J. Cochrane Database Syst Rev 2006 Jan 25; (1): CD005593 - Cholinesterase Inhibitors for Alzheimer's Disease." *Psychoneuro*, vol. 32, no. 11, 2006, pp. 508–508., doi:10.1055/s-2006-956993.

Bloomberg.com, Bloomberg, www.bloomberg.com/quicktake/drug-prices.

Clark, Amie. "Prescription Drug Prices and Costs." *The Senior List*, The Senior List, 3 May 2019, www.theseniorlist.com/medication/costs/.

Cully, Jeffrey A., and Melinda A. Stanley. "Assessment and Treatment of Anxiety in Later Life." *Handbook of Emotional Disorders in Later Life*, 2008, pp. 233–256., doi:10.1093/med:psych/9780198569459.003.0010.

Culo, Sandi, et al. "Treating Neuropsychiatric Symptoms in Dementia With Lewy Bodies." *Alzheimer Disease & Associated Disorders*, vol. 24, no. 4, 2010, pp. 360–364., doi:10.1097/wad.0b013e3181e6a4d7.

"Depression Basics." *National Institute of Mental Health*, U.S. Department of Health and Human Services, www.nimh.nih.gov/health/publications/depression/index.shtml.

"Elderly Nutrition 101: 10 Foods To Keep You Healthy." *Aging.com*, www.aging.com/elderly-nutrition-101-10-foods-to-keep-you-healthy/.

"Feeding Strategies in Dementia." *INDI Irish Nutrition Dietetic Institute*, www.indi.ie/fact-sheets/fact-sheets-on-nutrition-for-older-people/516-feeding-strategies-in-dementia.html.

Gale, Seth A., et al. "Dementia." *The American Journal of Medicine*, vol. 131, no. 10, 2018, pp. 1161–1169., doi:10.1016/j.amjmed.2018.01.022.

"Global Aging." *National Institute on Aging*, U.S. Department of Health and Human Services, www.nia.nih.gov/research/dbsr/global-aging.

Grande, Giulia, et al. "Physical Activity Reduces the Risk of Dementia in Mild Cognitive Impairment Subjects: A Cohort Study." *Journal of Alzheimer's Disease*, vol. 39, no. 4, 2014, pp. 833–839., doi:10.3233/jad-131808.

"Home Page." *Home Page*, www.socialworkers.org/.

"Home." *Anxiety and Depression Association of America, ADAA*, www.adaa.org/.

"How to Change Adult Diapers With Poop in Them | How To Adult." *LIVESTRONG.COM*, Leaf Group, www.livestrong.com/article/182806-how-to-change-adult-diapers-with-poop-in-them/.

"How to Get Prescription Drug Coverage." *Medicare*, www.medicare.gov/drug-coverage-part-d/how-to-get-drug-coverage.

"Importance of Taking Medications Correctly." *a Place for Mom*, www.aplaceformom.com/planning-and-advice/articles/importance-of-taking-medications.

Institute. "The Physical-and Psychological-Effects of Urinary Incontinence on Older Adults." *IOA Blog*, 28 Apr. 2017, www.blog.ioaging.org/medical-concerns/physical-psychological-effects-urinary-incontinence-older-adults/

Karageorgiou, Elissaios, and Bruce Miller. "Frontotemporal Lobar Degeneration: A Clinical Approach." *Seminars in Neurology*, vol. 34, no. 02, 2014, pp. 189–201., doi:10.1055/s-0034-1381735.

Kessler, Ronald C. "Lifetime and 12-Month Prevalence of DSM-III-R Psychiatric Disorders in the United States." *Archives of General Psychiatry*, vol. 51, no. 1, 1994, p. 8., doi:10.1001/archpsyc.1994.03950010008002.

Lambiase, Maya J., et al. "Prospective Study of Anxiety and Incident Stroke." *Stroke*, vol. 45, no. 2, 2014, pp. 438–443., doi:10.1161/strokeaha.113.003741.

Larsen, Dana. "Grooming and Hygiene Guide for the Elderly." *Senior Assisted Living Guides: Find Senior Care A Place for Mom*, 13 Aug. 2018, www.aplaceformom.com/blog/3-21-16-grooming-hygiene-guide-for-the-elderly/.

"Mary C. Mayo, MD." *Mary C. Mayo, MD : Neurology - Santa Monica, California*, www.uclahealth.org/reagan/mary-mayo.

"Mayo Clinic." *Mayo Clinic*, Mayo Foundation for Medical Education and Research, www.mayoclinic.org/.

Mccann, Heather, et al. "α-Synucleinopathy Phenotypes." *Parkinsonism & Related Disorders*, vol. 20, 2014, doi:10.1016/s1353-8020(13)70017-8.

Medscape Log In, www.reference.medscape.com/features/slideshow/falls-in-the-elderly#page=1.

Mendez, Mario F. "Early-Onset Alzheimer Disease." *Neurologic Clinics*, vol. 35, no. 2, 2017, pp. 263–281., doi:10.1016/j.ncl.2017.01.005.

"Multidisciplinary Teams Knock Down Barriers to Medication Treatment for OUD." *Home | Psychiatry.org*, www.psychiatry.org/.

"National Alliance on Mental Illness." *NAMI*, www.nami.org/.

"National Center for Injury Prevention and Control - Home Page|Injury Center|CDC." *Centers for Disease Control and Prevention*, Centers for Disease Control and Prevention, 16 Dec. 2019, www.cdc.gov/injury/index.html.

Prince, Martin, et al. "The Global Prevalence of Dementia: A Systematic Review and Metaanalysis." *Alzheimer's & Dementia*, vol. 9, no. 1, 2013, doi:10.1016/j.jalz.2012.11.007.

Ravi, U. "7 Common Health Risks of a Bedridden Patient." *PatientsEngage*, 30 July 2017, www.patientsengage.com/conditions/7-common-health-risks-bedridden-patient.

Reams, Nicole, et al. "A Clinical Approach to the Diagnosis of Traumatic Encephalopathy Syndrome." *JAMA Neurology*, vol. 73, no. 6, 2016, p. 743., doi:10.1001/jamaneurol.2015.5015.

Rockwood, K., et al. "Prevalence and Outcomes of Vascular Cognitive Impairment." *Neurology*, vol. 54, no. 2, 2000, pp. 447–447., doi:10.1212/wnl.54.2.447.

Rosenberg, Paul B., et al. "The Association of Neuropsychiatric Symptoms in MCI With Incident Dementia and Alzheimer Disease." *American Journal of Geriatric Psychiatry*, 2012, p. 1., doi:10.1097/jgp.0b013e318252e41a.

Roux, Hillary Le, et al. "Age at Onset of Generalized Anxiety Disorder in Older Adults." *The American Journal of Geriatric Psychiatry*, vol. 13, no. 1, 2005, pp. 23–30., doi:10.1097/00019442-200501000-00005.

Singh, Balwinder, et al. "Association of Mediterranean Diet with Mild Cognitive Impairment and Alzheimer's Disease: A Systematic Review and Meta-Analysis." *Journal of Alzheimer's Disease*, vol. 39, no. 2, 2014, pp. 271–282., doi:10.3233/jad-130830.

Stephenson, Joan. "Preventing Falls in Elderly Persons." *Jama*, vol. 288, no. 6, 2002, p. 689., doi:10.1001/jama.288.6.689-jwm20008-3-1.

Tan, Chen-Chen, et al. "Efficacy and Safety of Donepezil, Galantamine, Rivastigmine, and Memantine for the Treatment of Alzheimer's Disease: A Systematic Review and Meta-Analysis." *Journal of Alzheimer's Disease*, vol. 41, no. 2, 2014, pp. 615–631., doi:10.3233/jad-132690.

Truschel, Jessica. "Depression Definition and DSM-5 Diagnostic Criteria." *Psycom.net - Mental Health Treatment Resource Since 1986*, www.psycom.net/depression-definition-dsm-5-diagnostic-criteria/.

Tully, Phillip J., et al. "A Review of the Affects of Worry and Generalized Anxiety Disorder upon Cardiovascular Health and Coronary Heart Disease." *Psychology, Health & Medicine*, vol. 18, no. 6, 2013, pp. 627–644., doi:10.1080/13548506.2012.749355.

Vyrostek, Sara B., et al. "Surveillance for Fatal and Nonfatal Injuries--United States, 2001." *PsycEXTRA Dataset*, 2004, doi:10.1037/e307172005-001.

Wang, Gang, et al. "Reader Response: Diagnosis and Management of Dementia with Lewy Bodies: Fourth Consensus Report of the DLB Consortium." *Neurology*, vol. 90, no. 6, 2018, doi:10.1212/wnl.0000000000004918.

"What Is BvFTD? (Behavioral Variant Frontotemporal Degeneration)." *AFTD*, www.theaftd.org/what-is-ftd/behavioral-variant-ftd-bvftd/.

"What Is Dementia? Symptoms, Types, and Diagnosis." *National Institute on Aging*, U.S. Department of Health and Human Services, www.nia.nih.gov/health/what-dementia-symptoms-types-and-diagnosis.

What Is Psychotherapy?, www.psychiatry.org/patients-families/psychotherapy.

Zaccai, Julia, et al. "A Systematic Review of Prevalence and Incidence Studies of Dementia with Lewy Bodies." *Age and Ageing*, vol. 34, no. 6, 2005, pp. 561–566., doi:10.1093/ageing/afi190.

Made in the USA
San Bernardino, CA
20 February 2020

64761301R00084